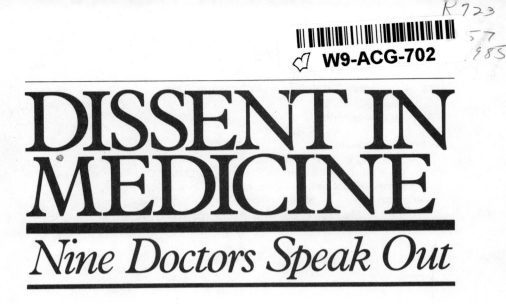

DISSENT IN MEDICINE

Nine Doctors Speak Out

THE NEW MEDICAL FOUNDATION

CONTEMPORARY
BOOKS, INC.
CHICAGO

Library of Congress Cataloging in Publication Data

Main entry under title:

Dissent in medicine.

Based on a conference held in Chicago, in Oct. 1984.
1. Medicine—Philosophy—Congresses. 2. Medical
errors—Congresses. I. New Medical Foundation (Chicago,
III.) [DNLM: 1. Medicine—congresses. WB 100 D616]
R723.D57 1985 610 85-10347
ISBN 0-8092-5265-1

Copyright © 1985 by The New Medical Foundation
All rights reserved
Published by Contemporary Books, Inc.
180 North Michigan Avenue, Chicago, Illinois 60601
Manufactured in the United States of America
Library of Congress Catalog Card Number: 85-10347
International Standard Book Number: 0-8092-5265-1

Published simultaneously in Canada by Beaverbooks, Ltd.
195 Allstate Parkway, Valleywood Business Park
Markham, Ontario L3R 4T8 Canada

CONTENTS

OPENING REMARKS*

Mr. Chatz: My name is James Chatz. I'm chairman of the New Medical Foundation. This is our first in what we hope to be many "Dissent in Medicine" seminars. My personal thanks to Dr. Robert Mendelsohn. The idea for this program came on a nice Saturday afternoon when we were sitting in the backyard deciding what the Foundation should do before the end of 1984. It was Bob's idea to put this program together. I thank him, and I thank all the participants for giving up their time to participate and prepare.

The New Medical Foundation was formed in the late 1970s. It is a tax-exempt foundation to support innovative forms of medical education for the public and the medical profession. It has limited resources, but we think it fills the gap in medical education, medical research, and the dissemination of what we call "the other point of view." Since the Foundation's inception, Bob Mendelsohn has been the president. Its Board of Directors consists of State Senator William Marovitz; Professor John McKnight; Professor Nathaniel Stampfer; Marian Tompson; and Dr. Jay Schmidt. Funds have been used in the past to support the

---

*The *Dissent in Medicine* meeting upon which this book is based took place October 1 and 2 in Chicago.

Alternative Birth Crisis Coalition, *The Journal of Child and Family*, and the American College of Home Obstetrics. In the immediate future, we have plans to support medical and public education, specifically in iatrogenic (doctor-produced) diseases. [See page 182.]

If you have any comments or any thoughts about this program, please let us know. We want to improve. We want to do it again. We would like your active participation in our future endeavors. At this point, it is my privilege to introduce the co-sponsor of this program, the president of Columbia College, Mike Alexandroff.

Mr. Alexandroff: It is my pleasure and honor to welcome the distinguished members of our panels and our guests to this unusual occasion which gives a platform to dissenting views of medical practice. As sponsors, our exclusive intent is to encourage informed public discussion of certain medical practices and to give the public a responsible opportunity to recognize controversy about these issues which are probably only representative of many other controversies in the medical sciences. For, after all, it is individuals of the general public who are inevitably affected crucially by medical enterprises. Certainly a healthy life is the paramount human concern, and its beneficiaries are increasingly identified as consumers and its practitioners as dispensers.

A vulgárity of language reduces the critical issues of health and medicine to matters of ordinary goods and services—and thus they become susceptible to conventional measures of profitability and privileged systems. The consequence of such diminished valuation is that concern for the physical environment, health care, and medical practice loses the priority, public understanding, and sense of human entitlement that would be paramount in an enlightened society. Moreover, in our rushing preoccupations with a high-tech consumer economy and our corresponding failure to separate health and medicine from ordinary measures, we foster a technical elite in medicine and in sciences who concentrate principally on products, processes, impersonal cures, and statistical exhibits. And the discussion of these is cast in credentials and a special vocabulary which discourages even an elementary understanding and an informed choice of treatment by those upon whom the medical sciences are practiced.

It follows that seldom, if ever, is discussion of medical interventions and practices publicly accessible. Instruction in healthy living and an informed basis for public consideration of the health science issues have little presence in the schools and are mainly absent in the lives of adult citizens, excepting brief moments of media interest in and publicity about radical cures and untested remedies. The process which leads to the physician's choice of treatment and prescription of medication is unavailable to public estimate.

And what influences, for example, do pharmaceutical detail men, the advertisements of lobbies and drug companies, the editors of medical journals, the manufacturers of medical equipment, the partisans of particular treatment, the major medical organizations, in medical schools, and the industries who profit from the health process have on the practice of health care and the creation of a safe, human environment? The answer, I submit, is exhibited in the failure of the nation to enact a comprehensive public system of support for universal health and medical care, in the failure to act decisively on conditions which sicken and fatally poison the environment, in the failure of governmental agencies to give the public genuine protection, and in society's failure to remedy the conditions of poverty and ignorance that culture human suffering.

Nowhere is there a subject which more deserves public discussion. And this rare platform for responsible dissent in medicine uniquely serves a critical human purpose. It is an occasion which gathers a panel of distinguished and leading members of the medical profession. It is a project not to endorse any particular idea or form of medical practice but only to encourage informed public discussion of the state and direction of the medical sciences and to give opportunity to hear and estimate the diversity of views which customarily are largely reserved for private forums. Undoubtedly many among us and within the medical profession have valid dissent from the views of the dissenters here. And so we hope our effort here will encourage widest public debate and perform as an early model of citizen participation in discussions of the medical sciences.

HOW MUCH SCIENCE IS THERE IN MODERN MEDICINE

A Dissenting View

Robert S. Mendelsohn, M.D.

INTRODUCTION OF THE SPEAKER

Robert S. Mendelsohn, M.D., is President of the New Medical Foundation, a nonprofit organization whose purpose is to encourage and support innovative forms of medical education. A practicing pediatrician for nearly 30 years, Dr. Mendelsohn presently maintains a general practice in Evanston, Illinois.

He served for 12 years as Associate Professor in the Department of Pediatrics, Preventive Medicine, and Community Health at the University of Illinois Abraham Lincoln School of Medicine. Previously he was an Instructor in Pediatrics at Northwestern University Medical School and taught at Loyola University's School of Education. He is former Director of Development at Michael Reese Hospital, and former National Director of Project Head Start's medical consultation service.

Dr. Mendelsohn received both his bachelor's and medical degrees from the University of Chicago and did postgraduate work at the Chicago Institute for Psychoanalysis. He is a diplomate of the American Board of Pediatrics.

He is the author of three best-selling books, *Confessions of a Medical*

Heretic, Male Practice: How Doctors Manipulate Women, and most recently *How to Raise a Healthy Child . . . in Spite of Your Doctor.* He writes a syndicated newspaper column as well as a monthly subscription newsletter, "The People's Doctor."

LECTURE

Dr. Mendelsohn: Jimmy Chatz told you the idea for this meeting was developed when we sat on our front lawns one day. Actually it goes back a little further than that. It began when my good friend Dr. Samuel Epstein pointed out to me with great emotion that the citizens of this country were not being told the truth about the dangers of chemical pollution of the environment. He discussed methods that we might use to further disseminate the other, the darker, side of the story. After that, Dr. Ed Pinckney of Los Angeles talked to me about the same situation in medical testing. He pointed out that 50 percent of all the medical costs in this country are spent on medical tests which are often useless and frequently dangerous. He felt that this information was not getting across to people. Then Jimmy Chatz and I started to talk and we came up with this idea of a conference called "Dissent in Medicine." Our original idea was to collect a group of doctors. Then we asked—why should we talk to ourselves? Why not invite other doctors, particularly those holding different views. (And I should point out that we dissenters dissent among ourselves, as well as from other doctors.)

We then decided that we should not restrict the discussion to ourselves and other doctors. Perhaps we should invite the press. That's when I called on Mort Kaplan, my good friend for many years. Mort did the public relations for this event without charge. (As Jimmy pointed out, The New Medical Foundation is a very modest institution.) Through Mort's help in establishing the PR, we have an unexpectedly large turn-out from the media. We then decided that, in addition to inviting the media, why not invite the public, since a number of people came to us and said, "Why can't we come?" (We invited the public at a different fee schedule from that of the professionals.) That's how this meeting developed.

To our knowledge, this is the first of its kind. There has never been a meeting of so many dissenters in medicine. Many medical institutions seem to be able to tolerate one dissenter. But no one has gathered them together in the same room. I know some of the doctors personally; others

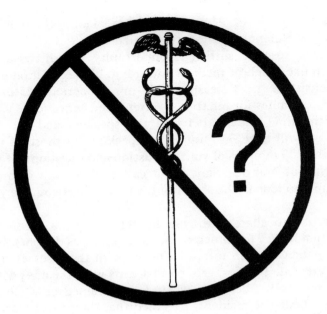

I know through distinguished members of their families. For example, Dr. Henry Heimlich and I met only yesterday. But his wife, noted journalist Jane Heimlich, is the author of the excellent book, *Homeopathic Remedies for the Home*. She and I have met at a number of meetings previously.

Out of the nine physicians here, seven of them came at their own expense. Mort Kaplan approached Mike Alexandroff, and Columbia College became a co-sponsor of this meeting. Hedy Ratner has ably served as conference coordinator. Among many responsibilities, she designed the striking logo on our posters. The logo consists of the caduceus, the symbol of medicine, overlaid by the international symbol for "Do Not Enter." We are very grateful to Hedy for that imaginative and creative idea. I have long felt that medicine is a religion. All religions have their own distinctive symbols. For example, my religion uses a six-pointed star; the Christian religion has the cross. The Religion of Modern Medicine has the caduceus. Perhaps some of you don't know the meaning of one of the components of the caduceus. The rod is the staff of either Mercury or Hermes (depending on whether you accept Greek or Roman mythology). Mercury was the God of Commerce, Eloquence, Cleverness, and Thievery. Hermes was the God of Science and Cunning—and the guide of departed souls to Hades. So much for the symbols of the Religion of Modern Medicine.

We decided to give sufficient opportunity for discussion at this meeting—unlike much of medical education. The education of medical students consists in great measure of 50-minute periods: 45 minutes for the lecture, 5 minutes for questions—often bogus questions. We decided to divide the time equally between the speakers and the audience. Therefore we will have 30 minutes of speaking by those of us on the panel and then 30 minutes of your discussion and questions. If you wish, you can write out your questions or you can speak directly from the floor. There's a microphone in the center of the floor. We encourage you to use it.

I would like to share with you how I became a medical heretic (assuming that heresy has much the same meaning as dissent). In the late 1960s, my patients began to return to me with the diseases that I had previously created. The first group of patients were the ones with cancer of the thyroid gland, because, when I was trained at Michael Reese Hospital as a pediatric resident, I learned that the proper treatment for tonsillitis was X-ray therapy. Together with hundreds of other doctors, I prescribed X rays for the tonsils. This led to an epidemic of tens of thousands of cases of thyroid cancer. The second group of patients had permanently yellow-green stained teeth from tetracycline given for the treatment of acne. The third group were the DES sons and daughters. When I was a medical student at the University of Chicago, I participated in the DES experiments in which we gave women that female sex hormone diethylstilbestrol in a fruitless attempt to prevent miscarriages. It didn't work, but it did leave us a generation of sons and daughters with tumors and malformations of the reproductive organs.

(I might point out that the sexism inherent in modern medicine is well exemplified by the differing recommendations for the treatment of the DES sons and the DES daughters. When the DES daughters first appeared with cancer of the vagina at very young ages, at 20 and 25 years of age, the recommendation was total vaginectomy. When the DES sons appeared with tumors of the testis, the recommendation was careful dissection of the tumor leaving the testis intact. The Religion of Modern Medicine is much more dangerous for women than it is for men because women make seven times as many visits to the doctor as men. Therefore, they are much more likely to be damaged.)

When I first recognized those events in the late 1960s, I thought that perhaps that was all past history in medicine. Doctors today must have learned from their mistakes. They certainly weren't going to repeat them over and over again.

But, when I look today at diagnostic ultrasound, immunizations, environmental pollution, amniocentesis, hospital deliveries, allergy treatment, and practically everything else in medicine, it is obvious that doctors haven't changed at all. They are simply making a different, new set of mistakes. The problem in medicine is not technology; the problem is one of ethics. The doctor has been trained since his earliest days in medical school not to share full information with the public. He learns that if you tell the public the truth about the drugs that are being prescribed, the people will not take those drugs. Of course he's right. When the government first mandated that the prescribing infomation for the birth control pill be included in each package, the sales of the Pill dropped by 30 percent. When Barbara Gordon wrote her best-selling book, *I'm Dancing as Fast as I Can*, showing the hazards of Valium addiction, the sales of Valium dropped by 40 percent. The Religion of Modern Medicine—and its doctors—have a different set of ethics than the rest of us. We have been trained that honesty is the best policy, but medicine doesn't believe that. That is the reason I've developed a deep respect for those dissenters in medicine who are ready to tell the truth to the public.

Our next speaker, Dr. George Crile, played an important part in my development. As a medical student I learned about Dr. Crile through his writings against radical mastectomy in the 1940s. Dr. Crile was the first to teach me by his example that if you have something important to say—and if doctors won't listen—go right to the press. In medical school, I learned the catechism of the Religion of Modern Medicine. When asked a question by a patient, the proper response is "just trust me,"or—to a female patient—"just trust me, dear." When faced with a patient who offers information different from that you gave him, the proper response is—"What medical school did you go to?" When faced with an older person—"What do you expect at your age?" When trying to sell a hysterectomy—"What do you need your uterus for? It's just a sack for cancer." Or—one of my all-time favorites—"We're taking out the baby carriage but leaving in the playpen." Doctors have strange ways of speaking—"Mr. Smith suffered a negative patient outcome": That means he died. Doctors have strange ways of thinking. The impact of medical education is so powerful that we doctors develop different thinking patterns from the rest of the population.

Valium, the number one all-time best-selling drug, carries as its

indications tension, anxiety, fatigue, depressive symptoms, acute agita-
tion, tremor, hallucinosis, skeletal muscle spasm, and spasticity. Its side
effects include fatigue, depression, confusion, tremor, hyperexcited
states, anxiety, hallucinations, and increased muscle spasticity. That
poses problems. If I prescribe Valium and it doesn't work, do I double
the dose or discontinue the drug? In addition, Valium is a very
interesting drug in terms of sexism because 80 percent of the Valium
prescriptions are written for women. Apparently doctors believe that
women are born with a congenital Valium deficiency that only they, the
doctors, can relieve!

Here is a report from the *AMA News* regarding testimony that Senator
Ted Kennedy gave before a congressional investigating committee. The
senator described a serious shoulder injury that he had suffered while
skiing in Vermont as a youth. His father, Joe Kennedy, took him to four
orthopedic surgeons. Three of them said he should be operated on. The
fourth said to leave it alone. The senator then demonstrated that,
following his father's choice of the fourth physician, the shoulder had
healed completely all by itself. At this point, the investigating committee
called on the AMA representative, Dr. Lawrence Weed, Chairman of the
Department of Medicine, University of Vermont Medical School. Dr.
Weed suggested the senator's shoulder probably would have healed just
as satisfactorily if the operation had been performed. You can't get that
kind of thinking in ordinary places.

In her book *Men Who Control Women's Bodies*, Diana Scully reports
that Dr. James C. Burt, a gynecologist in Dayton, Ohio, has designed a
surgical procedure that he calls "love surgery" and that he alleges
increases women's orgasmic potential. As Burt sees it, women are
prevented from being totally orgasmic because the anatomical design of
the vagina is faulty.

(That's just one of God's little mistakes. The Religion of Modern
Medicine assumes that God has made many errors. Obstetricians with
their 25 percent and rising rate of cesarean sections seem convinced that
God made a mistake when he didn't put a zipper into women's bellies.
Pediatricians, despite their lip service to breast feeding, seem convinced
that God made a mistake when he didn't put Similac or Enfamil into
women's breasts.)

Dr. Burt has his own feelings about God's mistakes. As Burt sees it,
the clitoris is not accessible enough to penile stimulation during inter-
course, thus causing "structural coital inadequacy" in the human female.
Now, once you have a diagnosis, you must intervene—so of course he

does. To compensate for this inadequacy, Dr. Burt has designed an operation termed "the Mark II vagina." For about $1,500, women can purchase the Mark II, which consists of lengthening the existing vagina by severing the pubococcygeal muscle (that's the muscle that holds up the bladder; if you cut that muscle, you then set up the woman later in life for urinary incontinence) in order to create a new set of female genitalia in which the vaginal opening has now been moved closer to the clitoris. According to Burt, some 4,000 women have had this surgery. Many of these operations were done experimentally during other surgical procedures without women's knowledge.

Another example of the bizarre thinking of doctors can be seen from doctor's strikes, in which doctors provide the only worthwhile part of medicine—emergency care, that 10 percent dealing with shock, trauma, hemorrhage, broken bones, spinal meningitis, and acute abdominal conditions. Could it be that the rest of medicine is either dangerous or, at best, unproven? Whenever doctors strike, throughout the world, the same result occurs: The mortality rate drops. The first strike was in Saskatchewan, Canada, in the late sixties. The second was in Los Angeles, where, according to Professor Milton Roemer of UCLA's School of Public Health, the mortality rate during that strike dropped by 17 percent. The third strike was in Columbia, South America, where the mortality rate dropped by 37 percent.

The fourth, and my favorite, strike was in Israel when, during an 85-day strike, the mortality rate dropped by 50 percent. This greatly concerned the morticians, who did a study of their own. They discovered the last time the mortality rate dropped that low was 20 years previously at the time of the last doctors' strike. The most revealing aspect of this strike was the doctors' thinking. The president of the Israeli Medical Society was asked to explain this drop in mortality. His answer was that since we doctors only responded to emergency cases and weren't bothered with the mundane, trivial complaints of our everyday patients, we were able to invest our best energies into the area of the truly critically ill and therefore save more lives. Isn't that a perfect reason for a perpetual doctors' strike? I noticed that in a more recent doctors' strike in Israel the doctors decided not to stop working. Instead, they went on a hunger strike in an attempt, I presume, to elicit the sympathy of the Jewish mothers.

Finally, what is the effect of modern medicine on the treatment of chronic disease, particularly—although not exclusively—cancer. In these fields almost all of modern medical treatment is unproven. The late

Morris Fishbein, M.D., editor-in-chief of the *Journal of the American Medical Association*, in his 1948 lectures on medical quackery to the medical students at the University of Chicago, myself included, gave the three criteria for quack medicine: (1) having unproven remedies, (2) being highly expensive, and (3) being widely publicized.

How well that definition fits most of modern medicine. For example, no form of cancer chemotherapy has ever been subjected to controlled scientific study, that is, in which half the candidates for therapy receive the treatment and the other half do not. Oncologists feel that such an experiment would be unethical. They believe so strongly in their treatment that they will not withhold it from a single patient. However, they do not consider unethical the exposure of patients to unproven chemical treatments that can kill them.

Doctors rely on so-called "historical" controls. They boast to patients that leukemia used to be 95 percent fatal 50 years ago and now, because of treatment, it is only 50 percent fatal. But they don't tell their patients that the concept of historical controls is anathema to true science. (I learned science from the legendary Dr. Ajax Carlson of the Department of Physiology and Medicine at the University of Chicago. In his Scandinavian accent, Prof. Carlson repeatedly challenged the students with "Vat iss the effidence?" Scientists know that diseases come and go. Today we have new diseases: AIDS, herpes, toxic shock, Legionnaires' disease. Old diseases, like scarlet fever and rheumatic fever, have either practically disappeared or dramatically decreased in virulence without any help from doctors. The only controls that count in medicine are contemporaneous controls.)

Every patient should therefore ask three questions of a cancer specialist who threatens him or her with chemotherapy or radiation or surgery. The first question is, "Doctor, do all your patients follow your advice?" Of course the doctor's answer must be no, since no doctor enjoys a 100 percent compliance rate. The second question is, "Doctor, what happens to the patients who don't follow your advice?" His answer must be, "We don't know, since doctors don't follow patients who reject their advice." (That's one of the rules in medicine—we follow up only on patients who accept our advice.) The third question is, "In that case, doctor, how do you know that the patients who reject your advice don't out-survive the ones who accept your advice?" Since the doctor doesn't know the answer to this crucial question, the only conclusion is that the most dangerous form of cancer quackery today is that which is inside modern medicine.

People ask me, "Dr. Mendelsohn, what do you think of laetrile?" My answer is, I think laetrile is marvelous because it keeps people away from doctors who will give them chemotherapy. They ask me, "Dr. Mendelsohn, what do you think of copper bracelets for arthritis?" (The late Mayor Richard Daley of Chicago wore a copper bracelet. When I would appear with him, he would often turn to me and say, "Doc, what do you think of my copper bracelet?" I would reply, "Does it work?" He would say, "Yes, it does." I would say, "Well, I think it's great." Then he would start his speech with, "The good doctor says. . . .") I love copper bracelets because they keep people away from rheumatologists who will give them Motrin, Butazolidin, Tolectin, or even kill them with Oraflex, the antiarthritic that had to be removed from the market last year.

What is my opinion on chelation? I cherish chelation therapy because it keeps people away from surgeons who will give them a coronary bypass or a carotid artery operation. Doctors complain that quacks keep patients away from orthodox medicine. I cheer! Since all the treatments, both orthodox and alternative, for cancer, coronary heart disease, hypertension, stroke, and arthritis, are equally unproven, why would a sane patient choose treatment that can kill the patient?

There is little chance for change in the near future. Proponents of alternatives believe just as strongly in their remedies as orthodox doctors in theirs. Therefore, both groups will continue to shun scientific, controlled studies. The only proven factor in orthodox therapies are the adverse reactions. Doctors not only admit this, but are proud. According to Eli Lilly, head of the drug company which bears his name, "Any drug without toxic effects is not a drug at all." Therefore, given the lack of science in all therapies, orthodox and alternative, present and future, what's a person to do? The obvious answer is to attend meetings like this, and to listen to the media, because the media today represent the most important avenue of health education to the public.

Thanks to the media, last year, people learned that four major drugs had to be removed from the market: Eli Lilly's antiarthritic Oraflex; Johnson & Johnson's pain killer Zomax; the drug used for morning sickness in women for 25 years, Bendectin (notice how that drug was named to sound like a blessing, a benediction—in reality it turned out to be a curse); and high-dose Marcaine, the major drug used for epidural anesthesia in women in labor. Thanks to the media, people now know that the American Medical Association is in agreement with me in opposing routine annual medical examinations. The American Cancer Society is in agreement with me in now opposing the routine annual pap smear. The American College of Radiology has now banned the routine annual chest X ray, and my own organization, the American Academy of Pediatrics, is now opposed to the routine annual tuberculin skin test and the routine X ray of children admitted to hospitals. So, I think that we are making great progress.

Thanks to the media, the people now know that a National Institute of Health consensus committee has warned every pregnant woman in this country that she should be careful when her doctor recommends diagnostic ultrasound. She should make sure that her doctor has a good reason for making that recommendation. And in the last four or five weeks, also brought to public attention by the media, Connaught Laboratories discontinued the distribution of their DPT infant vaccines. Ten or 15 years ago, there were 17 companies manufacturing DPT vaccines. Last year, there were only two because of the high rate of malpractice suits and the multimillion-dollar awards to the victims of vaccine damage. Wyeth withdrew from the market, leaving only Lederle and Connaught. Connaught's withdrawal now leaves only Lederle. I recommend that people listen to their own doctor, but always check out everything that he or she says. In medicine today, there is very, very little science. There is plenty of "clinical impression," which means we're guessing.

QUESTION AND ANSWER PERIOD

Q: My name is Henry Seifer, D.D.S., from Chicago. I have a few comments. I'm going to try to be brief. I feel privileged this morning to be in the presence of this distinguished panel. I must tell you that you were very honest, because I have found in my experience, the last 23 years, that I tried to have the medical profession give us an alternative. It's been absolutely a very, very big challenge. Now, let me just briefly give you a personal history. I have a daughter who when four years old was subjected, because of tonsillitis, to deep X-ray therapy. Four years later, she developed carcinoma of the thyroid. Now, that's devastating to any parent. I was on the telephone for 24 hours calling every thyroid specialist in the country to find out what course of treatment is best. Most of them said radical surgery, removing the sternocleidomastoid muscle. I finally reached a dear man, who's sitting on your panel, Dr. George Crile from Cleveland, and that's where I went. That was 30 years ago; he did not take out the sternocleidomastoid; he did a modified radical and, thank God, she's a mother today. She's an R.N. with a master's degree and has two children.

My wife was in perfect health and at age 57, going through menopause, was given estrogen. Two years later, she died of cancer of the breast. I attribute that truly to the estrogen. She was in excellent health before that. My brother was a very hypertensive individual and for years was given sedatives, tranquilizers, Valium, and the like and at age 62 died of cancer of the pancreas. My father, nobody telling him about it at that time (they just learned in the medical profession in the last decade that smoking is harmful), was a heavy smoker, meat and potato eater, overweight, and died at the age of 64. So you can see that the medical profession did not increase their life expectancy.

Now, I at the age of 46—that was 23, 24 years ago—started developing a deterioration of the complete digestive system, and I was treated for two years with antispastic drugs, sedatives, and so forth. They diagnosed it tentatively as Crohn's disease. Finally, after two years, they said they had to go in for a bowel resection with a colostomy and they gave me very little hope; they said maybe a year of life at most. And I said no, I'm leaving the medical profession because I feel they're perpetrating a fraud without money and my family and all of the people because they are protected by law to commit manslaughter. That's what I found in my experience and with God's help, some miracle (and that's a story in itself), I found a health-building system, and the health-building system reversed the pathology. I did not have the resection, I'm still here 23 years later, and the two doctors that were treating me are no longer alive, having become deceased in their 60s. Now, how did I do that? That's what I want you people to understand—that there is a health-building system. It means proper nutrition, food that is not contaminated with all of the chemicals that we find today. It means learning mental poise, for nobody has taught us how to deal with stress, we don't know that; we have to go out and learn it, either through self-hypnosis or transcendental meditation or yoga or some other form of dealing with stress, proper exercise, and mainly the detoxification program. How does one get rid of the toxins in our body? Through fasting—that's how I reversed the disease. I fast every year, and I want you people to understand I appreciate what you're saying, and you're saying a lot of things that are negative about the medical profession, but I'd like to hear ultimately what the *positive* approach is, what is good nutrition, what is good exercise? How do we detoxify, how do we learn mental poise? We've got something to learn, because right now, you've got your heads on the block. What I'm saying is, you're dealing with a great power structure, you're dealing with billions of dollars involved, and so there is a big thing ahead and we've got to work together.

Dr. Mendelsohn: Henry, thank you very much. Of course, you are aware that nutrition is not part of the Religion of Modern Medicine. Doctors believe in better living through chemistry. If you don't believe me, all you have to do is to ask a doctor, "Doctor, what should I eat?" He will say to you, "Just eat a well-balanced diet." If you want to find out what a doctor thinks a well-balanced diet is, just look at hospital food. Particularly in my specialty, the pediatricians seem obsessed with Jello. I have never been able to understand why they pour that junk food down the throats of poor, ill, defenseless babies. Now that they've been caught using Jello, they're turning to a new trick. They now prescribe Gatorade, the drink used for athletes, without telling people that Gatorade contains a number of chemicals, among them yellow dye number 5. Thank you very much.

While I believe in the importance of freedom, I must confess that I have certain reservations about freedom of choice. In the best of all possible worlds (which means if I had my way), nobody would be allowed to have back surgery unless they had prior mandatory consultation with a chiropractor. In the best of all possible worlds, nobody would ever be allowed to undergo cancer surgery unless they had prior mandatory consultation with a nutritionist. Nobody would be allowed to have an elective C-section unless they had prior mandatory consultation with a midwife.

Q: I'm John Barcardi, M.D. Mention was made during your comments, Dr. Mendelsohn, and also during the introduction that there needs to be a cooperative, concerted effort, rather an affirmative effort, to correct the deficiency that we find in modern medicine today. But what I have discovered as a parent of five children is that the state is becoming more and more involved in the area of medicine. My constant argument with the law is in relation to the immunization program that children must have to attend school. Now, I know there will be time for immunization questions tomorrow, but I'd like to raise the issue.

Dr. Mendelsohn: Before Professor McKnight begins moderating the next segment of the meeting, I have four references that I recommend for your consideration. I believe these books are among the best examples of documentation regarding the lack of science in medicine. The first is authored by journalists William Broad and Nicholas Wade, whom some of you may recognize as the ace writers for the publication *Science*. The name of the book is *Betrayers of the Truth: Fraud and Deceit in the Halls of Science*. It begins with Mendel and Galileo and proceeds right up to modern times telling us about the "fudge factor" in scientific research. The second, by journalist Martin White, is named *Health Shock: How to Avoid Ineffective and Hazardous Medical Treatment*, published by Spectrum. The third is an Australian book called *Medicine Out of Control: The Anatomy of a Malignant Technology*, by Richard Taylor. The fourth book, called to my attention by McKnight, is called *The Structure of Scientific Revolutions*, by Thomas S. Kuhn. I am now happy to turn the meeting over to Professor John McKnight.

INTRODUCTION OF THE FIRST MODERATOR

Dr. Mendelsohn: Our first moderator will be John McKnight, Acting Director of the Center for Urban Affairs and Professor of Communication Studies and Urban Affairs at Northwestern University and a friend of mine for more than 20 years.

Since joining the Center for Urban Affairs in 1969, John has been associated with many of its major research projects, including community health, urban disinvestment and metropolitan government, deinstitutionalized child welfare services, police anti-crime programs, and the effects of the perception of crime upon community responses. At present he is project director of the study of urban determinants of health and is a lecturer and consultant in social service delivery systems, health policy, community organization, neighborhood policy, and institutional racism with community groups, government agencies, and international agencies. Professor McKnight serves on the boards of directors of the Better Government Association, Business and Professional People for the Public Interest, and the People's Medical Society. Before joining Northwestern, he directed the Midwest Office of the U.S. Commission on Civil Rights.

I began my relationship with John and his wife, Geri, when I took care of their children when they were babies. In introducing John, I want to share with you one of his most distinctive epigrammatic one-liners, for which John is famous. This is one I like the most. It's when he talks about "helping professionals." John says, "A criminal stands a better chance at rehabilitation if he's never apprehended, a student stands a better chance of getting educated if he never matriculates, and a patient stands a better chance of recovering if he is never diagnosed."

TREATMENT FOR SOME CANCERS

A Dissenting View

George Crile, M.D.

INTRODUCTION OF THE SPEAKER

Mr. McKnight: Bob Mendelsohn and I probably met first over an examining table when he was checking my children, and I remember him in those days as being a physician who was a believer in the allopathic way of life. He would always say about his advice on our children, "We believe," and I've always been impressed by doctors who will say that to you: "We believe." I think it's a very important way of understanding what you are hearing because very often that is exactly what you're hearing; you're hearing about a *belief*. I have been impressed, knowing Bob Mendelsohn in the last 20 years, with his self-education and, while I think he learned the faith of allopathic medicine in medical school, it has been wonderful to watch him slowly but surely move into the realm of science. We get together several times a month, and I have noticed that in the last five years, when I hear him talking and I watch the way he's thinking, that I am now out of medicine, I'm not hearing somebody who's talking about medicine; I'm hearing somebody who has the kind of understanding and sense of inquiry that is the base of scientific revolutions. And I would recommend to you all the book by Thomas Kuhn, *The Structure of Scientific Revolutions*.

When Bob Mendelsohn asked if I would come and moderate a session, I was very pleased to do that because I come from an urban research center where we're concerned about the determinants of health in cities and I want to associate myself with his serious effort to ask the basic, and too often unasked, questions upon which the belief system called allopathic medicine is based.

Our first speaker today is a person who literally needs no introduction, Dr. George Crile. I was raised in little towns in Ohio, and when I was a kid they would talk about Dr. Crile's Cleveland Clinic with awe. In fact, I think that, in our view in Ohio, the Cleveland Clinic was the place one went before going to Lourdes. It was the place where the possibilities were known and best defined. Dr. Crile is a graduate of Yale College and Harvard Medical School. For 35 years, he led the Department of Surgery at the Cleveland Clinic and is the Emeritus Consultant there now. But I think everyone knows that in some basic way he is the spirit of the Cleveland Clinic. He's written hundreds of scientific papers and a dozen books, one of which, interestingly enough, is called *A Naturalistic View of Man*. His research on the utility, or nonutility, I suppose, of radical mastectomy resulted, I understand, in his being censured at one time by a medical society. Only in recent years has that censure been rescinded when the belief system finally came to grips with the scientific system.

I think that there is one thing that not many of you know about Dr. Crile, and you should, because it may be his most important talent. I am drawing here from one of his writings. It is in the *Crile Cornball Collection of Fiction, Fact, and Fantasy*, a poem called "Change Our National Emblem":

Give me a vulture, he's got my kind of culture.
He's kind and he's patient and true.
He's not like an eagle, a killer that's regal.
A buzzard will never harm you.

A buzzard's best business is livers and kidneys of something that's
    already dead.
He's never attracted by creatures still active. He waits and he uses his
    head.

That magnificent eagle we all hold so regal
Will kill any creature alive.
So give me a vulture with my kind of culture,
I want to be patient and thrive.

And he has. Dr. Crile.

LECTURE

Dr. Crile: Although Dr. Mendelsohn has asked me to speak on the subject of "Treatment for Some Cancers—A Dissenting View," I would like to speak also of some other areas of surgery in which I support views that are controversial. Because of these views my colleagues have often called me bad names and have accused me of endangering the lives and the welfare of patients. But gradually, in most of these areas, the test of time seems to favor conservatism. Whether because they are convinced that radical treatment is no longer necessary or because an enlightened public has begun to seek out the surgeons who were less radical, whatever the cause, radical mastectomy is on its deathbed, tonsillectomy is moribund, and circumcision survives more as a ritual than as a therapy. With this introduction I would like to discuss first the treatment of some types of cancer and then to point out that there is merit to conservatism in the surgical treatment of nonmalignant diseases as well.

When Dr. Mendelsohn says, and I quote, "The entire field of orthodox oncology will disappear as chemotherapy, surgery, and radiation for cancer are revealed as fundamentally irrational and scientifically insupportable," I cannot believe he really means it. This statement implies that no treatment of cancer is ever effective and that there is no scientific basis for using any of the conventional treatments.

Although I don't agree with Dr. Mendelsohn, I think that through gross exaggeration he is making a point that is both valuable and partially true. The values of ultraradical surgery, of routine postoperative irradiation, and of adjuvant chemotherapy have been grossly exaggerated and oversold to the public. That does not mean that each of these does not have its place in the treatment of cancer; it means only that the indications for treatment and the extent of treatment have not yet been defined by controlled studies. Fortunately, as was the case in cancer of the breast, such controlled studies now are being done and when completed and properly publicized they will lead the oncologists willy nilly to abandon their too-radical treatments and to offer what the public has learned is right.

Before moving on to specific examples, I wish to make it clear that the reason that surgeons have been so slow to abandon treatments like radical mastectomy is not only because the radical operation commands a higher fee than a conservative one but also because, when radical mastectomy was the standard operation, a surgeon was criticized by his peers when he did less. Occasionally in such cases, the local cancer board made the surgeon bring a conservatively treated patient back to the operating room "to complete the operation." And all the time a lawyer was looking over the surgeon's shoulder trying to find an excuse to have his client sue the surgeon for failing to perform an operation that was up to "the standards of surgical practice." It is that, and the fact that surgeons are craftsmen who enjoy practicing their craft and are reluctant to abandon operations whose techniques they have perfected, that make it hard for surgeons to change.

I have spent my entire surgical life in the three years of my service in the Navy and at the Cleveland Clinic. In both of these everyone is salaried and it makes no difference to one's income whether he does few or many operations, small ones or big ones, and one is also protected by the institution against both lawsuits and the criticism of fee-for-service colleagues. It is small wonder that I have taken the easy path and spent my life in looking for the flaws that fee-for-service private practice has unwittingly built into the practice of surgery. Sooner or later I believe that in this country, as is the case in all other civilized nations, the majority of surgeons will work for salaries and for the pleasure of service. And now, to be more specific, I would like to list some of the types of cancer which I think are being overtreated and for which I foresee simpler forms of treatment.

Twenty-five years ago the radical head and neck surgeons were advocating routine radical neck dissection for the girls and young women who had papillary carcinoma of the thyroid. This, with a long vertical scar, removal of the sternomastoid muscle and sacrifice of the eleventh nerve causes severe deformity and sometimes disability in the patients so treated. For about 20 years they persisted in doing this, and then gave it up and began to use the nondeforming, modified radical effective neck dissection. But then another radical group, although accepting the modified neck dissection, began to urge that all patients with cancer of the thyroid be treated by total thyroidectomy. They cited the frequent multicentricity of thyroid cancer as the rationale for the radical operation, but failed to note that this multicentricity consisted of microscopic foci of in-situ cancer of the type that can be found if searched for in up to 20 percent of clinically normal thyroids and that these foci simply do not enlarge if the patient is given suppressive doses of thyroid. As a result of the eloquence of the radical school, however, and/or the fact that larger fees are paid for total than subtotal operations, many surgeons are advocating total thyroidectomy in spite of the fact that the incidence of hypoparathyroidism, vocal cord paralysis, tracheostomy, and operative fatality is much higher than after the subtotal operation. They are encouraged in this by the oncologists who believe that radioactive iodine should be used routinely after total ablation of the thyroid—thereby, in the large doses recommended, subjecting the patient to significant exposure to possibly carcinogenic radiation.

Everyone except the patient profits from performing total thyroidectomy and giving radioactive iodine. The cost is three times that of subtotal thyroidectomy followed by suppression by thyroid hormone. Perhaps with the advent of DRGs (diagnostic-related groups) more attention will be paid to the economic factors. There is no controlled study that has shown better survival of patients with papillary carcinoma treated routinely by total thyroidectomy and 131-Iodine than those treated by subtotal thyroidectomy, followed by suppression.

Cancer of the breast is of course the classic example of a cancer that for a full century was overtreated, first by operations that were unnecessarily radical, then by radiation that was given more often than indicated, and now, if I am not mistaken, by chemotherapy given too often and for too long. Radical mastectomy has been replaced by the modified operation or by partial mastectomy or by lumpectomy and radiation, and the trend persists toward saving the breast in an ever higher proportion of cases, averaging now, at the Cleveland Clinic, more than 70 percent. But it has taken us more than 60 years to accept the modified radical mastectomy that my father practiced 65 years ago and the local excisions that Sir Geoffrey Keynes, in England, was advocating in the 1930s. When there is no incentive to change, it takes a long time for a different idea to prevail.

Cancer of the rectum is another disease which has often been overtreated, inflicting unnecessary colostomies on the patients who contract it. When the cancer is larger and low lying, deeply ulcerating, or encircling the rectum, the rectum must indeed be sacrificed and the patient must live with a colostomy. But when the tumor is small, fungating instead of ulcerating, and is below the level of the reflection of the perineum, it can be destroyed by fulguration as effectively as it can by abdomino-perineal resection. Also, since in the type of tumor that is suitable for coagulation, nodes are rarely involved (if they are involved, most patients are not cured by even the most radical operations), and since the mortality rate of the radical operations in average hands is up to 10 percent compared to practically zero for coagulation or destruction of the tumor by local radiation through a special proctoscope, the mortality rate of the operation is greater than the improvement in survival afforded by removal of the nodes. The conservative operation is thus superior both in comfort to the patient and in survival. But still, the rectum-saving procedures are not widely practiced. Most cancers that are too low to be treated by a rectum-saving anterior resection still are being treated by abdominoperineal resection.

Adenocarcinoma of the pancreas is another controversial cancer that some surgeons treat routinely by radical removal of the pancreas and duodenum in all cases in which the tumor has not given rise to obvious metastases in the liver or on the peritoneum. This is an operation that has an average mortality rate of 30 percent. That is the proportion who die, right now, as the result of the operation. Other surgeons recognize that, even in those patients whose cancers seem localized and operable, only about 1 percent are permanently cured. Many of these surgeons—except in exceptional cases when the tumor is small and localized, the patient young and strong, or the tumor of an unusual, low-risk type—would prefer to treat the patient by simply joining the gallbladder to the bowel so as to relieve the obstruction of the biliary tract and relieve the jaundice. Again, when one calculates the risk of dying, right now, from the radical operation, against the only 1 percent chance of cure, it is clear that the conservative operation results in more person-years of survival than the radical operation. Most surgeons are beginning to be more conservative in their treatment of adenocarcinoma of the pancreas.

There are many other cancers whose treatment is controversial, such as cancer of the ovary, cancer of the testicle, and cancer of the prostate, but these are out of my field of personal experience. I would prefer to move on to the discussion of the treatment of some of the benign diseases.

In World War II, I was stationed for more than a year at the U.S. Naval Hospital in San Diego where I was in charge of the acute surgery. In that period more than 1,500 appendectomies were done—most of them for acute appendicitis. This was at a time when the fear of appendicitis was so great that even in the absence of any physician, medical corpsmen were being applauded for doing appendectomies in lonely submarines.

Our experience with acute appendicitis, in which many appendixes had ruptured, indicated that "rupture" of the appendix resulted in bacterial contamination of the peritoneum but not in fecal leakage. Penicillin had just become available and with the cooperation of Captain Fulton, the Chief of Surgery, we observed 50 consecutive patients whose clinical signs and symptoms made us quite sure that they had ruptured appendices. These we treated with massive doses of penicillin and no operation. None of these patients died of peritonitis. One had a fatal thrombosis of the entire portal system and eventually died of it, a complication that appendectomy could not have avoided. In all the rest, the diagnosis was confirmed by delayed operation, before the patients were sent back to duty. We were convinced that appendectomy was not a necessary or even an effective treatment for appendicitis if penicillin were available. Since that time, with more effective antibiotics, the indications for operation are even less. The only real problem is how to be sure that it really is appendicitis, and not something that demands surgical intervention. In any event, from the time appendectomy was introduced until the time that penicillin became available, the number of appendectomies done each year increased, and in almost direct proportion to the increase in the number of appendectomies there was an increase in the death rate from appendicitis per 100,000 people of the population. In spite of this, even today, few patients or doctors question the value of appendectomy. My position on this is as unpopular as Dr. Mendelsohn's is when, at a meeting of pediatricians, he warns against immunizations.

There are other operations that are greatly overdone, notably thyroidectomy for benign disease. Nodules of the thyroid are palpable in at least 10 percent of older people and death from cancer of the thyroid is so rare that if you ask audiences of 1,000 people if any one of them had ever lost a friend or relative from cancer of the thyroid, there is rarely a hand that goes up. Once in a while someone says yes, and then I ask him, "Did he die of the cancer or the operation?" Often it was from the operation that the patient died. Yet out come all the little nodules and the big nodular glands of thyroiditis and even, in spite of the availability of iodine, patients with the hyperthyroidism of Graves' disease still are being treated by operation. Of one thing I am certain, and that is that if the patient knew the risk of this operation and knew that the radiation from iodine gave no more radiation to the ovaries than an abdominal X ray and that the radiation received by the thyroid sterilized its cells so that they could no longer reproduce and give rise to a cancer, and if they knew that the thyroid deficiency induced by the treatment was completely correctable by taking a single pill a day—no patient, if he or she knew that, would accept surgery.

Now, as to the little thyroid nodules and the diffuse goiters of thyroiditis, there is no longer an excuse to routinely remove these in order to rule out the possibility of cancer. Needle biopsy now is so accurate that it is rarely necessary to remove benign nodules. Last year, for example, 47 percent of the thyroidectomies done at the Cleveland Clinic were for cancers and the rest for hyperplastic nodules which suggested the possibility of malignancy or for large goiters that needed to be removed. Yet as recently as 1978, Dr. Roger Foster in a survey based on the research of the Commission on Professional and Hospital Activities containing data on 24,108 thyroid operations found that 13 percent were for Graves' disease, 58 percent for benign nodules or goiter, 11 percent for thyroiditis, and only 7.2 percent for cancer. If Graves' disease had been treated by iodine and if needle biopsy had been used routinely to diagnose nodules and goiters, all of these operations for thyroiditis and at least 80 percent of those for goiters could have been avoided.

A similar overuse of surgery exists in the diagnosis and treatment of lumps in the breast. Cysts are still being removed surgically instead of being aspirated in the office, and because needle biopsy is not always used in the diagnosis of breast lumps there are some surgeons who do open surgical biopsies on almost all patients with nodules. In these, the incidence of cancer is perhaps only one in 10, whereas the incidence of cancer in the practice of a surgeon who uses needle biopsy may be as high as 50 percent. Interestingly, the aspiration of nodules really pays off because, in the case of the breast, a cyst that is aspirated is cured and does not refill. In the thyroid, too, many cysts are curable by aspiration.

There are a number of minor disorders that can be treated by extensive operations or by simple office procedures. Notable among these are pilonidal cysts. *Pilonidal* means hair-nest and it is the bundle of hair that accumulates under the skin between the coccyx and the anus as a result of the hair growing inward through the dilated pores that some people are born with in that region. To cure it, all that needs to be done is to remove the hair with a crochet hook, through a preexisting sinus or through a tiny incision made in the overlying skin at the site of the dimple. Then the hair must be shaved or depilated to keep it from growing back in. Yet, to this day, in spite of the fact that it has been known for more than half a century that the hair does not grow from follicles within the sinus but from the outside, surgeons persist in performing the conventional radical operation that removes all the skin and subcutaneous tissue of that area and requires the sliding of flaps and/or the grafting of skin to close.

Lipomas and sebaceous cysts often are overtreated. The little fatty tumors that lie under the skin, sometimes several or even dozens of them, do not have to be cut out like cancers and then sewed up. All that is needed for most of them is a little local anaesthetic in the skin, a little incision with a stab blade, a little spread of the incision with a hemostat, and then pressure, so that the fatty tumor is squeezed and pops out through the hole. The skin doesn't even need a suture. Wens on the scalp can be treated the same way, without shaving hair—just incising, dilating, squeezing out the contents, and then grasping the sac with the hemostat and pulling it out.

There are many more conditions in which conventional treatment represents overtreatment. Consider, for example, what arthroscopy has done for injuries of the knee, enabling the surgeon to remove the offending chips of cartilage without the necessity of anything but a peep-hole incision. The technical advances in medicine and surgery are proceeding at such a rate that many procedures become outdated before they can be established. That is why it is so valuable for the public, through meetings like this and through the voice of the media, to keep in touch with the progress of medical and surgical practice.

There is little incentive for the surgeon to abandon a favorite surgical procedure that he has learned to perform with skill, pleasure, and reward to adopt a new and lesser procedure that uses different principles and requires a whole new training. There is no great incentive for the surgeon to say to the patient, "No, your tumor seems to be localized, you don't conjunction with an excisional biopsy as the definitive treatment of cancer of the breast. Likewise, there is no incentive for the radiotherapist to say to the patient "No, your tumor seemed to be localized, you don't really need any further treatment." Yet the radiotherapists are becoming quite conservative and cannot often be accused of overtreating. It is the medical oncologists whose turn has come, and it is these that today we must watch closely until the long-range survival figures are available and we learn for sure where adjunctive chemotherapy increases survival when it is given not for metastatic cancer that is causing symptoms but as a prophylactic measure in patients who have cancer that as yet shows no sign of spread. If it cannot be shown to do so, there is no need for so many people to suffer such extensive side effects as they do now in the hope that chemotherapy might effect a cure.

QUESTION AND ANSWER PERIOD

Q: My name is Harris Coulter. I'm a medical writer and a medical historian. Your lecture is extremely interesting, Dr. Crile. I have a question of a general nature. I got the impression from everything you said that in medicine the group or the doctor who advocates an extreme measure has a psychological advantage over the group or the doctor who advocates the conservative measures.

Dr. Crile: A psychological advantage?

Q: A psychological advantage, yes, in the sense that the person who promises a lot, who says we have to do much more in order to be certain of our results, has a kind of a psychological edge over the doctor who says no, we're not that certain, we have to be moderate, we have to proceed cautiously. I'm wondering if that is a correct impression, and, if it is a correct impression, if you could comment on it. Are there, for instance, institutional pressures inside medicine which favor a more radical or more far-reaching approach to the treatment of illness than a more moderate one?

Dr. Crile: That's a good point. I think in the past that this has been true. In breast cancer, for example, there was a very strong pressure from within the profession against those people who were doing anything less than a radical mastectomy. I had a friend one time who did a modified radical mastectomy on an older lady in her late seventies who wasn't very well and the tumor board at the hospital made him take her back to surgery "to complete the operation," as they said, which meant removing the muscles. That is the type of thing which was believed like a religion, and it was a very unfortunate period. I don't think for a minute that most patients feel that they are not getting the best treatment just because it's not the most uncomfortable treatment. I think most patients are very glad to seek out the treatments which are less uncomfortable. It's from within the profession that the criticism comes. The same way for chemotherapy: If you don't send a patient for chemotherapy, you may get controversy among your colleagues.

Q: Then if you lose a patient, then you've done the best and it's accepted.

Dr. Crile: Exactly.

Q: If you go ahead and do a modified radical operation and you lose the patient, then you're going to get the flag. Now, how do you deal with that?

Dr. Crile: That's exactly what happened all these years. Well, by now, in the matter of the breast, there are enough controlled studies, most of which came from abroad, which indicate that it makes no difference. What people don't understand is that, in this disease of cancer, the battle is won or lost before the patient ever sees the doctor. The local disease of cancer of the breast never kills anybody. But if it has metastasized elsewhere distantly before the patient sees the doctor, there's no radical treatment that's going to help it; on the other hand, if it has not, almost any treatment that destroys a cancer, and that could be local excision or radiation or anything else, is going to be equally good. That is beginning to be appreciated now.

Q: I'm Maryann Napoli from the Center for Medical Consumers in New York. Dr. Crile, you went briefly over the issue that women with breast cancer are not being overtreated surgically anymore and now they are being overtreated with radiation and chemotherapy.

Dr. Crile: I said not in the country at large. In New York are they being surgically overtreated still.

Q: Oh, OK, that's the way I see it. Could you give me a handle on the appropriate use of radiation, for women, say, who opt for the breast-sparing procedure, and have lumpectomies. What is an appropriate use of radiation for women who go that route?

Dr. Crile: You're asking a question which will not be answered for at least five more years, because currently there is a national breast-cancer adjuvant study under the direction of Dr. Bernard Fisher comparing the survival of patients who have modified radical mastectomy with patients who have lumpectomy and radiation and with patients who have nothing but wide local excision. I have not seen these figures, but I understand that they are exactly what one would expect: that the incidence of local recurrence is significantly higher in the patients who have just the local operation without radiation, but that to date, as in all other studies of breast cancer, there is no significant difference in survival. Now, this is hearsay evidence, I cannot tell you for sure if that is true, but I believe that it is because practically every other study has come out the same, with no difference once the local disease is eradicated. There may even be local recurrences, but those can be easily treated when they're picked up early. Most of these operations were done with axillary dissection because since you're there you might as well do that and it does no harm to remove the nodes, at least to sample them, and it gives you an idea of whether or not radiation might be necessary because if the nodes are involved the incidence of local recurrence is much higher.

As far as I know, immunotherapy hasn't ever done any good in any of the genuine adult cancers, and so far as I know nutritional therapy is just as good for the growth of the cancer as it is for the growth of the patient. I have read reports but, until I see the controlled scientific trials, I will not believe them. I do not believe in nutrition as a treatment for cancer, but I think nutrition is great to *avoid* cancer.

Q: It is known that the body can cause cancer and, if the body can cause it, the body can reverse it.

Dr. Crile: Occasionally a cancer disappears spontaneously, but this is rare and unexplained.

Q: OK, there is a doctor in Philadelphia who had two operations. He was coming from the funeral of his father in New Jersey, who was buried for cancer, and picked up two hippies who told him about the macrobiotic diet to reverse cancer. This has been in the blabber-mouth papers, but it was not in our news media, because it seems like our news media is a pet of the AMA and the FDA and a few others. We, who believe in freedom of choice—right or wrong, we still should have freedom—we believe that all things should be given fair treatment. If some nice, little, thinking doctor discovers something and it works, he is immediately crucified by the medical society, especially doctors in California but in other parts of the country as well. There are cures being made now—let's not call them cures; actually they are reversals: Cancer can be reversed. Now, the criterion for a cure to modern medicine and the bandits that run the big cancer society is that, if you live five years you are cured, right?

Dr. Crile: Untrue. No sensible person ever made any such statement. My friend, you show me the controlled trial in which cracked almond-seed residue and such have been successfully used! They just don't work in controlled trials. The reports you refer to are opinionated, and I don't believe a word you say.

Q: I'd like to ask you how you feel about estrogen therapy.

Dr. Crile: I think it's all right; I don't think there's any proven connection between breast cancer and the use of estrogen in minimum doses, though estrogen does increase the incidence of cancer in the uterus. You don't want to use more than is absolutely necessary. Especially if a woman has had a hysterectomy, I don't think there's need for the cyclic use of estrogen. I think it would be much safer to take very small, continual doses, because the cyclic use of estrogen causes the cells to undergo atrophy and then undergo hypertrophy again and it makes for new cells and the danger is when the new cells are born, because the new cell might be a cancer cell. It would be a bad thing, though, if you have a thing like in situ cancer or a history of cancer in one breast—I wouldn't use estrogen then because, if you have a cancer in the other breast, too, it could stimulate its growth.

Q: Dr. Crile, I keep hearing you say there haven't been enough controlled studies on the treatment of cancer.

Dr. Crile: No, no, on the surgical treatment there are a great many, and on radiation treatment a great many. All of those are fine; it's the dietary treatment for which there are no controlled trials.

Q: The one statement that I'd like to make is that the only people that can do controlled studies are medical doctors, and, if the controlled study has not been done, then whose concern should that be?

Dr. Crile: I think, first of all, every single cancer cell is a direct descendant of a cell of your body. Now, all of these diets are very good for your body and I'm not opposed to diets; I think that they may, in many cases, have a salutary effect on keeping a person healthy and well. Now, to say that because this diet which is so good for your body would be bad and cause death of the cancer cell is, on the face of it, absurd. The cancer cell is a part of your body. You're nourishing the cancer cell by giving them these diets.

I have no reason to distrust anything that I've seen from the National Cancer Institute. I think you can trust their statistics. The way that the statistics are released to the public may be misleading, but the statistics themselves are true.

Q: My name is June Perboner. I don't like to announce the study that's being undertaken before the scientist has released his reports, but there is a study currently being undertaken by a renowned medical cancer researcher who has all the degrees that it's possible to have and all the awards that it's possible to have, and he has proven—and the results will not be announced perhaps for another year, the studies are continuing—that the enzyme therapies with nutrition are successful and a particular doctor's work showing 100 percent irrefutable proof coming forth within about a year confirming. . . .

Dr. Crile: In what type of cancer?

Q: I can't disclose the types. I know it includes pancreatic cancer; I don't know if it includes soft tumors, but it does include hard tumors.

Dr. Crile: If you're curing pancreatic cancer with dietary therapy . . .

Q: With enzymes.

Dr. Crile: . . . you will end up on the right-hand side of St. Peter.

Q: Well, it's coming through, and the reports will be coming through in about a year.

Dr. Crile: I'm delighted to hear it, but I don't believe it.

Q: I've spoken before, so I'll be very brief. I would like to say that I believe that chemotherapy and radiation depress the human beings' immune system to such an extent that they cannot fight off their cancers. I believe that diet, nutrition, and a belief in what you are doing help to detour further metastases.

Dr. Crile: I think there is a lot of truth to what you're saying, but you did not say how we get rid of the local cancer because the local cancer will not be controlled by diet, nor will diet stop it from metastasizing.

Q: May I make a comment? Sir, I'm living proof also that nutrition will help. Seven members of my family died of cancer, and all were treated medically, which turned me against it completely. After four years, I'm still here and I have not been cut or had chemotherapy or radiation—you won't get me near it—and my family members are gone.

Dr. Crile: Did you have cancer?

Q: Yes.

Dr. Crile: What kind?

Q: Breast, uterus, colon, and lung.

Dr. Crile: And have had no medical treatment, no surgical treatment.

Q: No, sir.

Dr. Crile: How long ago? I need a little more confirmation. Would you mind sending me the slides of those so-called cancers?

CLOSING REMARKS

Dr. Mendelsohn: I was very interested, Dr. Crile, in your comments about the presence in certain glands, like the thyroid, for example, of cells that look malignant under a microscope but do not metastasize in a malignant way. There may be a discrepancy between the cytologic appearance of the cells and their nonmalignant behavior. Surgeons tend to do needle biopsies of the prostate in older men without telling them that in a significant proportion of these men, say about 30 percent over the age of 50 and 50 percent over the age of 60, that the biopsy will yield malignant-looking cells which will never become malignant in reality. I think it's important for us to publicize that such patients run a risk from the surgeon who finds malignant cells and jumps to the conclusion that this represents a cancer that will become malignant in reality.

I also wish to express my gratitude for Dr. Crile's remarks about appendicitis. All of us can be skeptical now if we ever hear the surgeon say, "I caught your appendix just in time; otherwise it would have ruptured." Now we can tell that surgeon, that Dr. Crile has given us evidence that rupture of the appendix is not all that bad, with 49 survivals out of 50 patients. (The citation for that study is *Surgery, Gynecology & Obstetrics*, 1946–47.)

Regarding the media coverage of medical dissent, in many areas our side may be overrepresented. I'm sure that 30 years ago Dr. Crile was the only surgeon in the entire country who opposed radical operations for breast cancer. Yet he received a lot of publicity. The dissenting voices against immunization today, even though they are very few in number, are receiving quite a bit of media attention. I regard the media as our ally rather than as the enemy.

Dr. Crile has a very intimate link to us Chicagoans. His wife is Helga Sandburg, Carl Sandburg's daughter, an author in her own right. Their home contains what should become a national shrine—the Sandburg room.

Dr. Crile: One thing that Dr. Mendelsohn said, the reason I didn't talk about cancer of the prostate wasn't that I didn't know anything about it, but that I simply don't believe in its treatment other than by estrogen or palliatively with the transurethral resection, and that's why I never go to have my prostate examined.

Mr. McKnight: I'm sort of pleased with an idea that Dr. Crile has that I wanted to just lift up for view once again: that, to his mind, progress is doing *less*. We're finding that's true in an awful lot of areas. There was a time when one might have thought that was sort of an unAmerican idea, that progress is always doing *more*, but I hear a very important and unusual theme that somehow it could be that we would be ahead by being more conservative, by doing less.

ENVIRONMENTAL ISSUES IN MEDICINE

A Dissenting View

Samuel Epstein, M.D.

INTRODUCTION OF THE SPEAKER

Samuel S. Epstein, M.D., is Professor of Occupational and Environmental Medicine at the University of Illinois Medical Center, Chicago. He has been Chief of the Laboratories of Environmental Toxicology and Carcinogenesis at the Children's Cancer Research Foundation in Boston, Senior Research Associate in Pathology at Harvard Medical School, and Swetland Professor of Environmental Health and Human Ecology at Case Western Reserve University Medical School. A recognized international authority on toxic and carcinogenic hazards due to chemical pollutants, he is the author of more than 250 scientific publications and six books including *The Politics of Cancer*, published by Anchor Press, and coauthor of *Hazardous Waste in America*, published by Sierra Club Books. He has served as consultant to various congressional committees, federal agencies, organized labor, public interest and citizen activist groups, and is President of the Rachel Carson Trust.

LECTURE

Dr. Epstein: I propose to discuss illustrative problems of environmental pollution and to explain how those most critically affected—namely, the citizens of the United States—are basically excluded and disenfranchised from decision-making processes in relation to involuntary and unknowing exposure to toxic chemicals in air, water, food, and the workplace. These decisions are made generally by powerful groups and organizations, institutions over which citizens have little or no control.

Cancer is a useful paradigm of failed decision-making. Cancer is the only major killing disease in industrialized countries that is on the increase. Heart disease, on the other hand, has undergone in the last decade or so major decreases in mortality rates. Last year about 420,000 people died of cancer. One in four of us now gets cancer; one in five of us dies from it. Based on projections and analyses of current trends, it is clear that in the early future, one in three will develop invasive cancer while one in four of us will be dying from it. There is no question that a critical examination of the data, particularly over the last decade or so, makes it very clear that there have been major recent increases in the overall incidence and mortality of cancer.

Overall, during the last two decades, there has been an increase in cancer incidence rates of about 2 percent per annum and mortality by about 1 percent per annum. But when you examine particular population groups, you find that these figures substantially underestimate the reality. For instance, for people over the age of 65, rates of cancer are *much* higher. For blacks, of all ages, their rates are approximately twice those of whites. Similarly, for certain consumer subgroups, women who were told over the last two decades to take Premarin for treatment of so-called "postmenopausal problems" as estrogen replacement therapy, there have been epidemics of uterine cancer.

We are also seeing great increases in cancer among other groups of the "general public," particularly those who live close to major industries that handle toxic chemicals of a carcinogenic nature. Substantial data demonstrate that a very important factor in cancer is where you live. If you happen to live close to an industry that is processing carcinogens you will be breathing them in.

Perhaps even more important are the occupational subgroups. In 1978, a study released by expert authorities in three major federal agencies concluded that past and current exposure to carcinogens in the workplace will be responsible for up to 18–38 percent of all cancers in future decades. In other words, a high percentage of cancer in this country is caused by exposure to occupational carcinogens. For instance, we know from the National Institute of Occupational Safety and Health that at least 10 million workers are exposed full- or part-time to 11 "high-volume carcinogens," and also that in certain industries, the rate of cancer at a wide range of organ sites is five to ten times that of the general population.

Current failure to control the cancer epidemic must be viewed from societally broad perspectives. The twentieth century is a century of major threats to society, which stem from "runaway technology," a rapid growth of technology, in the hands of expert "idiot savants," engineers, and nuclear physicists, whose rate of progress has been so rapid that it has outstripped the capacity of social control mechanisms. One of these threats is the chemical industries' role in "carcinogenizing" our environment with a wide range of toxic and carcinogenic chemicals, thus contaminating our air, water, food, workplace and hazardous-waste dumps all over the country.

What has been the nature of the federal response to this cancer threat? There has been a massive abnegation of responsibility. Hundreds of thousands of Americans have died due to the policies of the government, particularly the National Cancer Institute (NCI). In 1970, a group of consultants from the cancer chemotherapy establishment representing the NCI, the American Cancer Society (ACS) and their academic lobbyists, approached the Senate and told them "We know how to cure cancer. Give us the money and we'll do the job. We've been able to put a man on the moon, but only with a massive infusion of money. Do the same for cancer, and we'll cure cancer." So, the Senate set up a national panel of consultants on the "Conquest of Cancer," and about a year later they launched the "National Cancer Program" to cure cancer.

What has happened since then? The budget of the NCI has escalated to approximately $1.8 billion per annum. The ACS also collects vast sums of money from the public for their programs. Thus has been perpetrated on the American public two gigantic hoaxes: (1) the treatment hoax and (2) the prevention hoax.

The response to cancer treatment is generally assessed on the basis of five-year survival rates. The official party line of the NCI and ACS is to claim that as five-year survival rates in the 1930s were 25 percent (only

25 percent of the people survived five years), and by the 1980s the figure had reached 50 percent, this means, they said, "we are winning the battle to cure cancer."

However, much of these improved survival rates was not a reflection of increased ability to treat and cure cancer, but of a general improvement in surgical techniques, besides developments in antibiotic therapy and blood transfusions.

As far as the claimed improvement in the 1980s is concerned, these claims do not take into account the following three factors: First of all, we now have earlier detection, especially for some slow growing cancers, such as breast cancer. Secondly, we have improved follow-up and registration for nonfatal cancers. Thirdly, there's an improved diagnosis for nonmalignant lesions, particularly of the prostate and the breast.

It is my considered view that there have been no major advances in the treatment of cancer particularly the major cancer killers—lung, breast, and colon. For decades, there have however been important advances for less common cancers, particularly childhood leukemias and Hodgkins Disease. However, if you can con the public, continue conning Congress that we are winning our battle against cancer, then this justifies continuing major budget increases.

Prevention is the second hoax. We know a great deal about cancer, particularly how to prevent it. We have plenty of information that would allow us to modify our environment to minimize exposure to chemical carcinogens in air, water, food and workplace. But, the reasons why such information is not exploited to advantage reflect a spectrum of economical and political constraints, apart from ignorance and indifference of the NCI and ACS, largely reflecting industry self-interest.

Not only have the NCI and ACS been unsupportive of legislation and regulation in the area of cancer prevention, but on many occasions leaders of these groups have actually trivialized the role of exposure to carcinogens in our environment. Instead, they have espoused strategies that have been perfected by the chemical industry, known as "blame the victim." In other words, if you get cancer, it's your own fault—you smoke too much, drink too much, you've chosen the wrong parents, you spend too much time in the sun. It's your fault and nobody else's fault. The NCI has enthusiastically funded programs in the blame-the-victim area. At the same time, it has steered away from recognizing the very important role of involuntary exposure to carcinogens in our environment and the workplace.

Faced with increasing public concern, the NCI is now claiming that it is spending one-third of its $1.8 billion budget on cancer prevention, which is untrue. The money it is spending on prevention goes into programs such as chemoprevention which wait for people to be exposed to carcinogens, and, in the time from exposure to carcinogens to the subsequent development of cancer, they try administration of chemicals and drugs in an attempt to see if they can modify the cancer, and others that are calculated to support the position of blaming the victim. And at the same time, the NCI has inflated its estimates as to what it is really spending on cancer prevention and has attempted to minimize its expenditures on cancer treatment.

So, over the past decade in particular, as the public tax dollar has gone to swell budgets of the NCI and ACS, these institutions have not only perpetrated a hoax about our ability to treat and cure cancer, but at the same time have fought hard against increasing attention to prevention. It is my view that what we need now is to take responsibility for policy-making in cancer prevention away from the institutionalized basis of the NCI and the ACS. Instead, decisions should be made with involvement of the citizens at large of this country who now demand that cancer prevention be a number-one priority.

Additionally we need a National Citizens' Commission to inquire into the failures of the NCI over the last decade and the failures of the ACS. We need to politicize this issue of failed cancer prevention and to remove it from the hallowed corridors of scientific authority.

Apart from such problems within the medical profession, or industry, there are even broader concerns, concerns of our runaway technology. Prior to the 1940s, the production of synthetic organic chemicals was minimal because such chemicals were manufactured with difficulty by the destructive distillation of wood and coal. In the early 1940s, however, with the advent of fractional distillation of petroleum, suddenly it became possible to synthesize and manufacture new chemicals clearly and on a large scale for any particular purpose. In 1940, this country synthesized and manufactured about a billion pounds of synthetic organic chemicals. By 1950, the figure had reached 30 billion, and by 1980, the figure had reached 450 billion pounds per annum of synthetic organic chemicals. The overwhelming majority of these chemicals has never been tested for ecological effects, let alone for chronic public health effects. In fact, it wasn't until 1976, with the advent of the Toxic Substance Control Act, that the administrator of the Environmental

Protection Agency (EPA) had the power to request industry for test data on such chemicals prior to their release to commerce.

The chemical industry fought tooth and nail to prevent such legislation, just as it has fought tooth and nail to prevent workers' right to know, and to prevent communities' right to know how they are being exposed to industrial carcinogens in air, water, food, workplace, and environment.

Overall, the testing program of the U.S. chemical industry is a joke. The National Academy of Science's National Research Council recently did an analysis of some 65,000 industrial chemicals and concluded that test data were available on a very small fraction of these. I remember having worked as an expert witness for the EPA in 1974 on the cancellation suspension of Chlordane and Heptachlor, two highly carcinogenic pesticides. In the course of this it became clear the Velsicol had suppressed information on their carcinogenicity. Senator Kennedy became interested in this whole matter and said, "Now let's take a look and see what's going on with the data base on pesticides." So, the data on 26 pesticides with the highest tolerances on common foods were examined. These are among the common contaminants all of us are exposed to which you don't know about because you're not informed; there's no labeling; there's no right to know. This investigation revealed that for 24 of these 26 pesticides, the data base was so grossly inadequate, that you couldn't express any opinion whatsoever on safety or hazard.

One of the areas of concern that has come to my attention in the last two decades as a consultant to congressional committees, working with the media, and with agencies, examining the data base of industries on a wide range of industrial chemicals and food additives, pesticides, drugs, and on the basis of a very careful analysis which has been published in detail in the *Politics of Cancer* is the conclusion that information developed or derived from individuals or institutions with economic interests in their outcome is suspect until proven otherwise. Suffice it to say that there are numerous examples which demonstrate that industry has frequently suppressed, manipulated or destroyed information pointing to the hazard of their products or more commonly just failed to test. This is commonplace. So, essentially what we're seeing now is the responsibility of a vast new 20th-century technology in the production of vast amounts of untested or hazardous synthetic materials for which we have no biological experience, with growing contamination of our air, water, food, and the workplace.

Many of such synthetic industrial chemicals are persistent, fat-soluble and bio-accumulated by factors of a million to a billionfold. At the same time, the public is being excluded from information concerning these chemicals on the grounds that toxicological data are proprietary. So, we are now faced with an anarchical situation in which industry has been allowed to run amok. On the basis of short-term benefits to industry, long-term hazards to the public and environment are being tolerated. You might say, "Well now, look, this is the price of progress. We're sitting here in an air-conditioned room, and, you know, a bit of cancer is the price we have to pay for progress."

That isn't true. Let me give you just a few examples. For instance, many times we are told by industry, "You need this material because, in its absence, production of food and fiber will suffer or industry or commerce will suffer." In fact, this is generally not the case. When you examine these claims carefully, you can demonstrate the existence of alternative technologies that are safe or safer. For instance, in the hazardous waste area, we have 180,000 industrial impoundments in the country—ponds, pits, and lagoons scattered over the country with toxic chemicals—due to the fact that industry has defecated its toxic detritus all over the countryside over the last few decades. There were other ways of coping with these wastes—very simple, safe methods, methods that would have saved industry money. Recycling and recovery are examples. Another case involves pesticides: many of those we use have no demonstrable efficacy. In 1973, I served as an expert witness for EPA at Aldrin-Dieldrin, highly carcinogenic pesticides, cancellation hearings, Shell was unable to produce evidence that these pesticides had any efficacy whatsoever, because for their major use, namely corn and soybeans, the affected insects had been demonstrated to be resistant for the prior decade or so. Everybody in this room has Aldrin and Dieldrin in his or her body fat. Did you ask for it to be there? No. Do you know it's there? No. Do you benefit from it? No. Does the farmer benefit from it? No. Who benefits from it? Shell does.

The same goes for ethylene dibromide. The idea that you need it as a fumigant is nonsense. In fact, simply by refrigerating fruit and vegetables from areas that have imported medflies for two days, you'll kill the insects very effectively.

Suffice it to say, it isn't an argument of progress vs. cancer. It's an argument against short-term economic benefits to industry and the disenfranchisement of the public and long-term risks of the public.

I would now like to turn to one serious threat of the future, food irradiation. Since the 1950s, the radiation industry has been trying to persuade the public and the government that they don't need safe food additives, pasteurization, refrigeration. Instead, "let's zap the material, and that will sterilize it."

There are three major uses of food irradiation using Cobalt 60 or Cesium 137 for gamma radiation. The first major use involves low dosages, less than 100 kilorads, for control of spoiling of fruit and of medfly, as also advocated by the FDA. Now, show a lemon or an orange that has been irradiated with a low dosage to a "simple housewife" who will immediately say, "Now look, the peel is blemished, there are little pockmarks on the peel or the pulp's mushy." She would be told by industry and the FDA, "Don't be concerned about that; we know better; we know this is perfectly safe; we know it doesn't alter the food." And furthermore, "we're not going to label the food that has been radiated because we don't want to increase your hysteria." That is exactly what Department of Health and Human Services secretary Margaret Heckler said in a 1984 public press conference when she announced that food irradiation was going to be introduced as an alternative to EDB. We needed EDB like a hole in the head; and we need food irradiation less still.

The second major use involves the medium-level dosage, 400–1,000 kilorads to reduce bacterial counts. This is already being approved by the FDA for spices. The third major use, high-level radiation, is the stuff that the food radiation industry really is looking forward to: zapping out over 1,000 kilorads to sterilize bacteria and viruses. This will be absolutely tremendous, they feel, for long-term treatment of most stored foods.

Now, let us see what kind of testing has been done over the last 30 years by the industry. The testing has simply involved taking irradiated food and feeding it to animals. When no apparent effect was seen; they said, "You see, it's fine." Now, a fundamental precept in carcinogenicity testing is that carcinogenicity tests in animals are very insensitive because a very small numbers of animals are tested compared to the very large human populations at risk. For instance, an average test is done with 50 to 60 animals, and the humans exposed may border in the millions. Therefore, assuming a carcinogenic effect in humans of one percent, .1 percent or .001 percent effect which can translate into many thousands of cancer deaths in this country, the chances of picking it up by testing animals at low levels, even assuming similar sensitivity in humans and animals, are close to nil, which is exactly what the industry wants.

In none of these studies on food irradiation has any attempt been made to test appropriate extracts of the food. We know that, when you irradiate food, you produce a wide range of what we call URPs (unique radiolytic products). These are stable, radiolytic products—peroxides, carbonyls, epoxides—that are poorly characterized but that generally fall into the class of carcinogens. There has been no attempt to extract and concentrate them, and feed them to animals. The FDA admits this should be done, but says it's difficult and, therefore, they don't want to go ahead with that.

Now, the objections to radiation are several. First of all, science aside, if somebody says, "We're not going to label it for you," you should be immediately suspicious. If you're told, "We're not going to tell you what foods are being irradiated or not," you should immediately be even more suspicious. The first scientific reason reflects the toxicologically uncharacterized nature of URPs. The second is the fact that radiation can induce bacterial resistance—among other things, botulinus resistance, and thus increase botulinus and food poisoning. The third, and a very important point, a series of studies have shown that irradiation can massively increase production of aflatoxin, which is a mycotoxin or fungal toxin that is highly carcinogenic in very small concentrations in parts per billion and is known to be responsible for high incidence of liver cancer in Africa.

Over and above this, there are major nutritional losses in irradiated food, especially with rice and other staples. Also there are major occupational hazards from the large-scale use of cobalt 60, especially when this is going to be entrusted to the poorly developed technological capacity of Mexicans to irradiate materials at the Mexican-American border before coming to this country. Also, this is going to result in a massive increase in the volume of radioactive products in commerce.

Now, that's just a little taste of what is happening, decisions that are being made behind closed doors by the cabal of industry interests and governmental linkages. But, disenfranchisement of the American public is the basic issue.

Talking about disenfranchisement of the American public leads to Wauconda, Illinois. What is happening in Wauconda now is a *very* important test case for what happens when, in a fundamentally demo-

cratic society such as ours, an individual or a group of individuals wishes
to exercise limited personal rights of free choice. Wauconda is a small
community about 50 miles northwest of Chicago that a few years ago was
concerned about problems of mosquito abatement. The town decided
that it was not going to allow mosquito abatement programs that would
swamp the areas and the waters with chemicals they knew nothing about,
and that could contaminate the local environment. They objected to the
programs on three grounds: (1) they raised questions of safety; (2) they
raised questions concerning expense; and (3) they asked if it really
worked. They got no satisfactory answers to any of these questions and
they went ahead and banned the mosquito abatement program. Here you
have a small group of councilpersons—men and women without scientific sophistication, but the essence of grass roots America, the Morton
Grove of America. These people, in February of 1984, said, "We are
concerned about the fact that pesticide companies come in and treat our
lawns with chemicals, with pesticides, and we don't know what they're
doing. Can't we do something about it?"

Now, before going on to tell you what they did about it, let me make
it clear that this just wasn't a group of hysterical ignoramuses. There are
somewhere in the region of 40,000 pesticide formulations, with approximately 1,000 active ingredients, 75 of which are manufactured by ten
large chemical companies. Every year, we use in this country about 1.3
billion pounds of pesticides, about 50 percent of which have agricultural
uses, and a substantial amount of the other 50 percent is used in homes,
lawns, gardens and urban programs. A soybean or corn farmer will use
about 2 pounds per acre. Do any of you have any idea how much
pesticide per acre is used on suburban lawns in Chicago? Up to about 10
pounds per acre. Now, included among these pesticides are pesticides
such as 2, 4-D, that have been clearly demonstrated to be teratogenic
(cause birth defects). For instance, in 1969, as chairman of a Panel on
Teratology of HEW Secretary Finch's Commission on Pesticides and
Their Relation to Environmental Health, we examined data on a wide
range of pesticides, and stated categorically as a unanimous conclusion
that herbicides such as 2,4-D, which have been clearly shown to be
teratogenic, should be restricted to prevent any human exposure. But the
lawn companies still use such hazardous pesticides.

Now, the "radicals" of Wauconda demanded the following: They said,
"After the pest control companies come in, we would like them to put a

little sign on the lawn telling people to stay off the lawn for 72 hours and naming the pesticide." The response of the chemical industry was, "How dare you ask what the name of the pesticide was?" First of all, this would frighten you; secondly, you wouldn't understand it; thirdly, you have no rights to it; fourthly, it's going to be expensive; and fifthly, if you go ahead, we'll sue you." That is exactly what they did. Sidley and Austin, one of the largest law firms in the world, with branches in Saudi Arabia, Hong Kong, Singapore, Europe, and based in Chicago, is now suing this little community that's had the temerity to say, "We want to know what chemicals you've been using." It wasn't even a question of informed consent. Wauconda didn't say to the pesticide people, "Please tell us what chemicals you are going to use before you spray." They simply said, "We would like to know, after you've used it, what you've used." This is preposterous, but this is a microcosm of the whole problem of technology running amok and past abnegation of responsibility by citizens in this country in the past, coupled with intimidation of citizen groups that now try to exercise minimal rights. If I were to have rewritten that Wauconda ordinance, I wouldn't have written anything like that. I would have said, "Before you come into our community, we want to know the name of the pesticides. We want to have toxicological data. We want to have written information. We want to know how much we're being exposed to. We want to know monitoring data. We want to know the health effects. We want to know why you're not using programs like integrated pest management control, as they are using in Berkeley. Why do you want to bring in these carcinogenic, teratogenic bio-accumulative agents into our environment with no alternatives?" That's the ordinance I would have written, not the modest milk-and-butter language that the Waucondans wrote. But the Waucondans are making a first stand, and I think we should all applaud them. At the same time, we should not just applaud them but find out from them how we can be of help, because this isn't a scientific or medical issue. This is a fundamental issue in democracy that transcends the "narrower" problems such as issues of cancer, birth defects.

I'd like to end by quoting, if I may, from a world-renowned American radical: "I hope we shall crush in its birth, the aristocracy of our monied corporations which dare already to challenge our government to a trial of strength and bid defiance to the laws of our country." (Thomas Jefferson, 1816.) Thank you.

QUESTION AND ANSWER PERIOD

Q: My name is Frank Netry from Toledo, Ohio, and I'd like to say that I'm very happy that the public was invited here today. I was involved in the medical industry for 10 years in the radiation field, and what appalled me was the blame-it-on-the-victim approach that the doctors took with us as medical workers. They were always worried about the patients' getting radiation, but it didn't seem to be of any consequence to us as workers. The doctors were always the first ones to leave the room in the event of the radiation being around.

Dr. Epstein: The same problem occurred with the atomic veterans. Whenever the major atomic blast went off, the higher echelons from the Atomic Energy Commission and the military always went below and put on protective garb. It's just the troops that were left above surface line.

Q: OK, you said 420,000 people were dying from cancer per year. What percentage of other subclinical and other diseases do you believe could be caused by environmental pollution?

Dr. Epstein: Well, I simply focused on cancer because the cancer data are the easiest and most accessible. When it comes to birth defects, we can't give national data because we don't have a national birth registry. I have no doubt that there are close associations between occupational parental exposure to a wide range of toxic chemicals in the workplace and teratogenic drugs that have been used indiscriminately in the past, and a wide range of birth defects. Also, pregnant women living in the vicinity of groundwater contaminated with teratogenic agents are of concern. So there are a very wide range of diseases, including birth defects, chronic respiratory disease, liver disease and kidney disease, that can be connected with occupational and environmental exposure. The associations between exposure to chlorinated hydrocarbon organic solvents of a wide range and liver and kidney disease are very clear-cut. However, I believe the point you're making, that cancer is only one part of a whole problem, is correct.

Q: One other short question. It's a major task for us to try to stop all these major companies. What do we do on an individual basis to detoxify ourselves, and what do you do personally as a detoxification program?

Dr. Epstein: I think the most important thing is to participate in the American democratic process and assert rights as a citizen. That is the fundamental issue, and that's the issue that we have failed miserably in. To a certain extent, this failure has been compounded by enthusiasms, and I'm not belittling this, of people in saying that, if they modify their own lifestyles, they'll be OK. There is no question whatsoever that anybody who smokes needs his head examined; however, it is equally clear that smoking isn't the only cause of lung cancer. There is a wide range of industrial causes of lung cancers, and the chemical industry is only too happy to use tobacco as a smoke screen to divert attention away from a wide range of occupational carcinogens. But, again, the prudent lifestyle is important. Clearly, the young man who goes to work in an industry and works with chemicals anonymously labeled AB-34 is in no way able to modify his lifestyle; he's exposed on an involuntary basis. If you drink water, you can't help it, basically. If you live downtown in a major metropolis, close to industry, everyday you will be inhaling substantial concentrations of toxic and carcinogenic chemicals. For instance, in Baton Rouge, Louisiana, in the heart of the petrochemical industry of the United States, where somewhere in the region of 60 percent of ethylene dicholride, the basic petrochemical feedstock is manufactured, concentrations of 25 or so carcinogenic chlorinated hydrocarbons—such as chloroform, carbon tetrachloride and trichloroethylene—are there in the downtown air, in concentrations from 5 to about 15 g/m³. This is not trivial. So, by all means, let us all jog, let us all not smoke. Let us all be moderate in our lifestyles, but this isn't where the action's at. The action is at failed democracy. This is what I'm here to talk about today.

Q: I'm Marjorie Fischer. I'm president of the Chicago chapter of the Human Ecology Action League, which is a national lay group that is concerned about medical effects of various environmental exposures. I have a few brochures for anyone who would be interested. I have just one comment. I want to very heartily thank Dr. Epstein for his support of the Wauconda people.

Dr. Crile: I just am very much impressed with everything you've said, Dr. Epstein, and I agree with everything except one very small thing. That is, on cancer, you say, no major advances have been made in treatment of cancer for 30 years, and in the cancers that affect adults, I think you're absolutely right. But in Hodgkin's disease, leukemia, lymphomas, Wilms' tumors and so forth, in children, I think you'd have to give credit.

Dr. Epstein: I couldn't agree with you any more, Dr. Crile. My comments about the absence of major advances refer to the major killing cancers, which are lung, breast, and colon. Dr. Crile is, of course, absolutely right. There have been dramatic improvements for Hodgkin's and childhood leukemias, particularly over the last decade. However, just a cautionary note: We are beginning to see more second cancers in these children, 10, 15 years later as a result of their apparently successful prolonged remissions from cancer chemotherapy. I strongly believe that there is a place for cancer chemotherapy, a limited role indeed, and in these areas that we talked about—childhood leukemia, Hodgkin's— chemotherapy and radiation do play great roles. But let us not lose sight of the fact that radiation is carcinogenic, and most chemotherapy treatments with alkylating agents are carcinogenic. However, if you or I had a child, the likelihood is that we would certainly say, "I'll take my chances, and I'll go for chemotherapy." However, when it comes to the poorly discriminate extension of chemotherapy in the NCI and ACS programs to a wide range of solid tumors for which there isn't impressive evidence that they do anything other than perpetuate the basis for claims for inflated budgets, I would suggest that a healthy dose of skepticism is *de rigeur*.

Dr. Mendelsohn: Well, if the two of you, Dr. Crile and Dr. Epstein, agree on something, it would take a fool to dissent, but dissent I must. Maybe as a result of my pediatric background, I'm a little more suspicious of the so-called advances in the treatment of children's cancers, primarily lymphomas, Hodgkin's, and leukemias, because I think there are a number of other possibilities. One of them is that the children's cancers have changed in composition. Now, I would suggest that even though nobody has ever looked into this, there must be a certain number of children's cancers that have resulted from the widespread radiation of our feet when we were children and we got our feet tested in that machine that left an indelible mark on my personality. Even today, when I go to a shoe store to get new shoes, I don't believe they really fit, because there's no X-ray machine. So, I'm suggesting that, as a result of the irradiation of our feet, the irradiation of our tonsils, the irradiation of our thymus glands, of our skin for acne, that we may have produced an epidemic today of leukemias and lymphomas that may not be the same as the kind that existed 30 or 40 years ago. And maybe, since we don't have any controlled study, because there are no studies in which half the patients, half the candidates for treatment, are not treated, it's possible that what we are really seeing is not the result of treatment, but rather the result of the natural course of doctor-produced disease.

I would also like to make the point, just in the interest of symmetry, that we are ending up this morning's program with a critique of the ACS by, I think, one of the most notable people in American medicine today, and we are going to begin this afternoon's program with a critique of the American Red Cross by Dr. Henry Heimlich. I'm sure we're all looking forward to that.

Also, I'd like to point out for those of you in the audience who may not be aware of it that Dr. Epstein's critique of the cancer statistics has found major support in the last two weeks. I'm referring to the September 16th article in the *New York Times* in which a number of statisticians made, I think, the same kinds of criticisms of the cancer establishment statistics that you heard today from Dr. Epstein.

Finally, I'd like to suggest a possible explanation for why we are not getting any farther in our actions as citizens, and I'd like your comments on this theory. If the doctors are the priests of our society, and if they are so involved in the creation of internal pollution in our bloodstreams every day, how can they speak out against external pollution? I think that that's why we are seeing the leadership of our society, the doctors, failing to exercise their responsibilities because, after all, if a doctor is going to talk about external pollution by chemical and other kinds of environmental pollutants, he then also has to talk about the dangers of diagnostic ultrasound. He has to talk about the dangers of the X rays. He has to talk about the dangers of all the chemicals used in the treatment of major diseases, and we cannot expect a doctor to do this. Therefore, maybe what we should really be doing, if we want to make it possible for people, for ordinary citizens, to achieve something effectively as citizens, we have to be exposed, we have to direct our fire at the doctors who are standing in the way of citizen activity against external pollution.

Dr. Epstein: I couldn't agree more. I don't think there's any question that there are a variety of reasons why the medical industry is not only indifferent but also hostile to citizen initiatives. One, of course, is the mind-set of scientific authority, or what we used to call in England, "Nanny knows best," which is the old English way of saying, "Leave it to authority." Now, of course, the traditional emphasis of medical industry on treatment as opposed to prevention is another fact. The medical establishment has, through history, been opposed to concepts of prevention. In fact, every major public health advance throughout the ages has been imposed upon the medical industry or profession by outsiders.

There is a wide range of factors involved, quite apart from ignorance and indifference, including the actual complicity of the medical establishment in industrial testing, in interpretation of epidemiological and toxicological data, acting as "over-loyal" doctors for industries, justifying the failure to test, failure to warn, failure to label. It's a complicated spectrum in which the factors you raise are very, important—the fact that the medical profession has clearly fought against rights to know and disclosure.

These are all parts of a complex scenario. When it comes to the question of childhood leukemia, I beg to differ with you. You say the childhood leukemias may be very different, the moon may be made of blue cheese, and I'm willing to listen to you tell me the moon is made of blue cheese if you offer me some basis for belief. However, the fact is this: We have information on childhood leukemias, on treated childhood leukemias, prior to the present, the modern chemotherapy era, and in different parts of the world now—some industrialized countries, some less industrialized countries—and I don't think there's any serious question about the fact that childhood leukemia is a fatal and a fairly rapidly fatal disease, depending on what particular variant.

To prove this in a way that would satisfy some critics would entail the following: One would take 500 children with leukemia. Two hundred fifty of these would not get treatment or would be treated with macrobiotics and what have you, and the other 250 would get the chemotherapy. Then we'd see what would happen. If you'd like your child to be one of the 250 that had macrobiotics, good luck to you, my friend. I wouldn't let mine. I don't want that kind of proof. I'm satisfied, and I would suggest that the serious evidence clearly demonstrates that this is one area in which there is proven evidence of the usefulness of chemotherapeutic drugs. It must be borne in mind, of course, that the usefulness isn't quite all that it's cracked up to be because some of these kids will go and get a second cancer from which they will die as a result of the treatment. But with that small caveat, I totally agree with you.

Q: My name is Beth Carpenter, I'm an RN and I'm also president of a coalition for pure water. I want to talk about fluoridation. As a nurse, I always thought that you had to have fluoride in your water to have good teeth. I started doing some research, found out from the EPA that they had no dumping zone for sodium fluoride because it was a usable, industrial by-product that was going into our public water supplies and into the toothpaste companies. Our public health officer has told our community that fluoridation is competely safe without any risks, and they also will not debate, scientifically debate the issue. I'd like to know your comments on fluoridation.

Dr. Epstein: I'm going to ask you a question, before I answer your question. Are you concerned about the fact that in groundwater all over the country we are now identifying a wide range of chlorinated hydrocarbon carcinogens, pesticides, trichloroethylene, dibromochloropropane, for which the evidence on toxicity, carcinogenicity, and teratogenicity are clear-cut, with no argument about them? Does your group have concerns for this, and are you doing anything on this?

Q: Well, yes, we'd like to, but first we'd like to fight fluoridation.

Dr. Epstein: I understand. Now, what I'm suggesting to you is the following: Here we have, with due respect, a lunatic situation in which we have in increasing areas of the country alarming data on the presence of highly toxic, highly carcinogenic materials, and there's no reasonable argument for their presence. We know that minimally, on a national level, 1 percent of all groundwater is contaminated with a wide range of pesticides and chlorinated hydrocarbons. And in some parts of the country this is even as high as 20 percent. You have well water in parts of the country, in Long Island, where levels of trichloroethylene approach the part per million level for which we not only have good animal data, but also some human data, including clusterings of leukemias. You have those substances for which the data are clear-cut, and you have the fluoride situation. I would, without going into a lot of technical discussion, submit to you that the question on fluoride is arguable. Now, not only is the question arguable, but the problem is made far worse by the link between the fluoridation people and the laetrile groups. So, you have on the one hand evidence of clear and unequivocal hazard to society for which your group, with due respect, doesn't seem to express great concerns. On the other hand you have the arguable fluoride situation. I'm not disputing some of the points you make. I'm all in favor of debate and would be more than happy to, if time permitted, discuss this in further detail. So, it is difficult to develop a high degree of enthusiasm for this problem, and it is difficult for me personally to place this on a high priority level. In one area I would agree with you, that this is an involuntary exposure and that, when it comes to involuntary exposures, the public, you and I, have as much right to say yea or nay as the next person. So, therefore, you have the fullest rights, in my view, to demand open debate, but I'm just very curious as to the basis for your priorities.

Q: I just have one question, Dr. Epstein. You said that the process should be politicized in order that the citizen get a voice in the issue. How would you advocate actually politicizing the making of scientfic decisions in these areas. Have you had any specific proposals?

Dr. Epstein: Well, I'm not really talking about science. I'm talking about the media. I'm talking about the fact that here we have a fundamental issue of the public being subject to involuntary exposures of a kind that they didn't ask for, that they had not given previous permission for, and for which there is, to say the least, excellent evidence of potential hazard if not real hazard. This is the fundamental question. When it comes to interpreting the details of the scientific data, I don't really think that's a great mystery. There have been so many expert committees, including governmental committees, that have made statements on interpreting carcinogenicity data, interpreting the significance of negative epidemiological data, and that isn't the problem. We need more information like a hole in the head. What we need is implementation of data already available. We have so much information on, for instance, how to dispose of hazardous waste safely, which we're not doing. We have so much information on involuntary exposure of workers to a wide range of toxic and carcinogenic agents in the workplace for which there's no argument. We're not implementing this information. It's a massive failure of implementation. It isn't a problem of shortage of scientific data; it's a political issue.

Professor McKnight: On that note, which was the one we began with, let me stress again the point that I think Dr. Epstein made so well, that in the kind of toxic environment that he's talking about it's very difficult for individuals to be successful in trying to live healthful lives. He says, after all, it's really a question of whether we can act as citizens, because in a toxic world, in a toxic environment, you can't really escape it alone. I take this occasion then, to make a little plug since this is the end of my moderatorship. About a year and a half ago, seven people, of which I am one, founded what we hope will be the first broad, national organization of people who are focused on the kinds of health problems that Dr. Epstein is talking about. It's called the People's Medical Society. We've had a phenomenal response, with about 70,000 people joining in the last year, and I was very pleased to hear Dr. Epstein talking about problems such as the proposition that toxicological data are not proprietary. I think this is one of the issues that we want to begin to focus on and take on.

Dr. Epstein: Just one very brief comment, if I may: You may be interested to hear of a Supreme Court decision, *EPA v. Monsanto*, I believe July 26, 1984, in which the United States Supreme Court ruled that the chemical industry has no rights to claim that toxicological data are proprietary, and that the public has to be given access to such data. Thank you.

Suggested References

Davis, D.L., et al. "Cancer Prevention: Assessing Causes, Exposures and Recent Trends in Mortality of U.S. Males, 1968–78," *Teratogenesis, Carcinogenesis, and Mutagenesis* 2: 105–135, 1982.

Epstein, S. S. *The Politics of Cancer*. New York: Anchor/Doubleday, 1979.

Epstein, S. S., and Swartz, J. B. "Fallacies of Life-Style Cancer Theories," *Nature* 289: 127–130, 1981.

Epstein, S. S., et al. *Science* 224: 660–666, 1984.

National Research Council. "Report of the Committee on Disposal of Hazardous Industrial Wastes." Washington, DC: National Academy Press, 1983.

Office of Technology Assessment. "Technologies and Management Strategies for Hazardous Wastes Control," Congress of the United States, March 1982.

Seidman, et al. "Probabilities of Eventually Developing or Dying of Cancer, U.S. 1985," *CA-A Cancer Journal for Clinicians* 35: 37–56, 1985.

National Research Council. "Toxicity Testing: Strategies to Determine Needs and Priorities," Washington, DC: National Academy Press, 1984.

INTRODUCTION OF THE SECOND MODERATOR

Dr. Mendelsohn: The moderator for this afternoon's session is Professor Hilmon Sorey of Northwestern University. Hilmon and I go back a long way because he was originally my boss back in 1971, when I was the head of the Pediatric Outpatient Department of Michael Reese Hospital and Hilmon Sorey was the administrator of the entire clinic, and he solved many problems for me. Professor Sorey received his MBA degree from the University of Chicago, and now Hilmon's title is Professor and Director of the Program in Hospital and Health Services Management of the Kellogg Graduate School of Management at Northwestern University. I'm proud to introduce to you Hilmon S. Sorey, Jr.

CHOKING, DROWNING, AND RESUSCITATION

Overcoming Twenty-Five Years of Medical Errors

Henry Heimlich, M.D.

INTRODUCTION OF THE SPEAKER

Professor Sorey: Thank you, Dr. Mendelsohn. Dr. Mendelsohn has been a longtime friend, mentor, and teacher. I still seek his advice, and I believe after this particular conference, I'll be a qualified dissenter. We've had some dissenting experiences all along. It even spills over into the hospital management side. I teach students who are being trained to enter the health services management field. Both Dr. Mendelsohn and Dr. Epstein serve as guest lecturers in my course "Introduction to the Health Services System." I'm very flattered to be invited by Dr. Mendelsohn and Mr. Chatz to participate in this program. I certainly have enjoyed this morning and feel confident that you're going to enjoy the speakers this afternoon. I congratulate the New Medical Foundation and Columbia College for sponsoring and undertaking this initiative.

Our first speaker this afternoon is Dr. Henry Heimlich, a world-renowned lecturer, scientist, author, researcher, medical leader, and television celebrity. Most of us know him as the physician who invented the "Heimlich Maneuver," a procedure which helps people to cough up food that gets stuck going down. This "Heimlich miracle," as it is called by some, also saves the lives of drowning persons by expelling water from the lungs. Dr. Heimlich lectures at universities, community meetings, corporate conferences, and national societies, in addition to television appearances, always with the aim of saving lives and improving the quality of life. One of his newest inventions is the Heimlich Micro Trach for the rehabilitation of emphysema patients. He has perfected the Heimlich valve, which saved hundreds of lives in Vietnam, and is widely used in civilian chest surgery and emergency facilities. His Patriots-for-Peace initiative has popular support from the media, world leaders, industrialists, and college students. Its purpose is to have public opinion press President Reagan and Soviet General Secretary Gorbachev for definitive answers to the question: "Why are the U.S. and the U.S.S.R. building for nuclear war?" World peace, Dr. Heimlich says, depends on seeking the cause of the conflict rather than on prolonged discussions on arms control.

Dr. Heimlich was educated at Cornell University, a surgical resident at Mt. Sinai and Bellevue Hospitals in New York City, and holds numerous honorary degrees. He is Professor of Advanced Clinical Sciences, Xavier University in Cincinnati, and President of the Heimlich Institute. He authored *Dr. Heimlich's Home Guide to Emergency Medical Situations* and also Created HELP, which stands for Dr. *H*enry's *E*mergency *L*essons for *P*eople, Emmy Award-winning one-minute animated television cartoons that teach medicine to children. Dr. Heimlich says, and I quote, "If everyone in the world placed his arms around someone else to learn to save a life, I believe there would be peace forever."

I am pleased to present to you Dr. Henry Heimlich, who will speak on "Choking, Drowning, and Resuscitation—Overcoming Twenty-Five Years of Medical Errors."

LECTURE

Dr. Heimlich: Thank you very much, Professor Sorey. I do want to first correct or dissent, if I may, from a statement made by Bob Mendelsohn this morning that the speakers are all dissenters. Bob, I am not a dissenter. You see, I know I'm right, and those who disagree with me are dissenters. It's sort of like people in the peace movement who feel they have to apologize even though they are right, whereas it is those who are building for war who are the stupid ones.

I'd like to first quickly run through the Heimlich Maneuver so we know what we're talking about. People often ask me how the name came about and this is the true story. The Maneuver was out about two or three months when I received a call from two editors of *JAMA*, the *Journal of the American Medical Association*. They said, "This technique has saved so many lives we're going to write a story on it in the medical news section of *JAMA*. We want to name the procedure for you, but don't know whether to call it the Heimlich Maneuver or the Heimlich Method; which do you prefer?" I answered, "Well, I'm thrilled and gratified that you're doing this, but you're the editors." They replied, "You see, a maneuver is something performed once, or you may repeat it, and it does its job; whereas a method is a sequence of steps, like a urine analysis." I said, "Maneuver!"

The Heimlich Maneuver is a technique for saving the life of a person choking on food or another object. It consists of external compression of the air in the lungs in order to provide a flow of air from the larynx sufficient to expel the obstructing object.

As a chest surgeon, I knew there would be enough air to accomplish this end; but it was necessary to prove through animal studies and subsequent research that it actually would work. The concept was to create a flood of air away from the lungs and toward the mouth. One of our studies actually measured the flows. The technique had to have a simple design because a mother has to save her child in four minutes, or there will be brain damage and death. Therefore, you can't go looking for an instrument. It had to be a hands-on procedure.

We found out we could generate a flow of 205 liters/minute by pressing upward on the diaphragm and that that was the safest, easiest method to use. We did not want to compress the chest; not only was it less effective, but you stood a danger of crushing the chest, as occurs with CPR (cardiopulmonary resuscitation).

We receive many reports and, just as any doctor loves his patients, I am very gratified by the pictures of children who were saved by their parents. These reports frequently lead to information which, in itself, provides knowledge about the Maneuver. A letter from a doctor who is the Director of Medical Services at Albert Einstein Medical Center in Philadelphia tells how his wife was sitting at a dinner party choking on a chicken bone, and by two applications of the Maneuver, the chicken bone, which was 1½ inches long and pointed at both ends, shot out of her mouth. The important thing about that was, as our studies showed, it's not necessarily the *pressure* effect that expels the choking object like a cork shooting out of a champagne bottle; even an object that does not completely block the airway, like a bone, can be ejected, because it is the *flow* of air, like the effect of squeezing a bellows, that expels an object.

We also learned from a woman who told how she was choking when she was alone. Choking on a piece of meat, she threw herself against a porch railing and saved herself. From that report and others we learned that people can save themselves. Another report advised that one could save himself by use of his own hands or by pressing the abdomen against an object such as the edge of a sink or the side of a table. What I would like to show by these reports is that you can learn an awful lot from your patients or, in this case, from people who wrote in to tell us of their experiences.

A news release from the AMA came out in 1975, a year after the Maneuver was first published. It stated that the Heimlich Maneuver was officially endorsed by the American Medical Association Commission on Emergency Medical Services and that it is approved as a means of saving lives. We felt this was rather unusual. That action set the Maneuver on the way.

Someone said to me last night, "What are you speaking at this meeting for? The Maneuver has been universally accepted by all organizations. What's your dissent?" It is not the Maneuver that I will be speaking about, but other factors in the treatment of choking, drowning, and resuscitation that are of importance.

By the way, the AMA came out again with a cartoon in the *AMA News*. A physician and a nurse are standing alongside a candy machine that is crushed. The doctor says "What happened to the candy machine?" The nurse answers, "It took my quarter for the fifth time and didn't give me any candy, so I gave it a Heimlich Maneuver."

I noticed last night that the Playboy Foundation had contributed to this meeting, so I feel it proper to refer to a *Playboy* cartoon. In it we see the husband in the doorway and another fellow kneeling on the floor nude with his arms around a similarly unclad lady, obviously the wife. The man on the floor says, "OK, ma'am, let's run through it once again. If a person is choking, you put your arms around their waist. . . ."

CHOKING

The historic background on choking was best reported by Dr. Milton Uhley of California (*Clinical Symposia*, 31: 24, 1979). He located a paper dated 1677, presented by Robert Hook at the Royal Society of London.

It reported on a man who, for colic, swallowed pistol shot, apparently a usual treatment at the time. One lead shot went into his lung. The important thing about this report from more than 300 years ago is that this man existed with this problem for a while, and when it got real bad he was hung upside down and was pounded on the back without result; he subsequently died. Pounding on the back and holding him upside down was proved to be of no benefit.

Dr. Uhley also cited a monumental paper by Samuel Gross published in 1854, whose studies described everything about foreign bodies in the airway that all doctors in the last 130 years have subsequently confirmed. Dr. Gross reviewed the case of a boy who aspirated a foreign body. Each time he was bent forward and hit on the back, he turn deeply cyanotic and lost consciousness and Gross realized that the object was sliding up against the vocal cords and blocking off the slit between the cords. He warned against turning anyone upside down who was choking. He also described how hitting on the back, in many instances, drives an object from the throat into the lung or trachea.

This finding was confirmed in repeated reports from the prestigious Chevalier Jackson Clinic in Philadelphia, which had experience with 6,000 foreign bodies in the lung or esophagus. The clinic emphasized that in many instances, when a person had been hit on the back, it drove an object down into the lungs or tighter into the glottis, cutting off the air supply. The clinic warned that if someone is choking, never hit him or her on the back because you can convert a partial obstruction of the airway into a fatal complete obstruction. Its reports extend from 1917 until the present time.

Dr. Gabriel Tucker, Chief of Pediatric Surgery at the Chicago Children's Hospital and Professor of Otolaryngology at Northwestern University, has emphasized in his writings that, should someone choke, do not hold him or her upside down for the reasons mentioned above and do not hit him or her on the back or the object will wedge tighter. He also states that putting your finger in a choking person's mouth can frequently push an object in tighter and this has caused many deaths. Professors B. Raymond Fink of Washington State University and Edward Patrick of Purdue University independently proved than when a choking person is hit on the back, the obstructing object can go down rather than loosen.

In 1982, Drs. Richard Day, Arthur Dubois, and Edmund Crelin of Yale University Medical School (Dr. Day is a former President of the

American Pediatric Society) published a very detailed study using advanced instrumentation *(Pediatrics,* 70: 113, 1982). They actually measured the forces resulting from backslaps and found that an object is driven *downward* at a force of 3 Gs, three times the force of gravity. They determined that if a person has an object in the throat and it is partially obstructing, if you hit him or her on the back, the object will become more tightly wedged. They pointed out that the forces followed Newton's law: To every action, there's an equal and opposite reaction. For example, when sitting in the front seat of a car that is hit from the rear, a person's head is driven backward.

Since 1933, the Red Cross has taught that you should slap people on the back if they are choking. There was no scientific basis for this recommendation; it was apparently an old wives' tale. The *Transactions of the American Bronchoesophageal Association* reported that the Association had warned the Red Cross in 1969 that their backslaps were killing people and wrote that the head of the Red Cross advised that he had changed the procedure. As a result, the Red Cross textbooks, from 1970 to 1979, on page 94 said, "Do not allow anyone to slap you on your back if you are choking and do not try to dislodge an object from another person's throat by this means except as a last desperate effort to save his life." For those ten years they were very much aware that hitting people on the back was an extremely dangerous method for treating choking.

We have reports of several hundred people endangered or killed by backslaps. The *Alabama Medical Association Newsletter* describes a case where a child was held upside down and hit on the back, and due to this delay progressed to loss of consciousness before the Heimlich Maneuver was applied and saved her.

In *Clinical Symposia* in 1979, I reported on the first 1,134 choking cases that had been documented as being saved by the Heimlich Maneuver. In 174 of those, backslaps were tried first, without success, and—this is the important thing—35 of these 174 choking victims *had fallen unconscious* before the Heimlich Maneuver was applied. That meant they were seconds from brain damage and death. That is firm documentation.

Speaking of 1,134 people is similar to talking about those killed in war who are faceless. What got me very much involved in exposing this problem of backslaps was a report from the Ohio State Department of Health of a two-year-old boy named Charles Tate of Dayton, Ohio. Charles's story, confirmed by the Ohio State Department of Health, was that he was held upside down and hit on his back by his uncle as he died from choking on an object. Another report was about Timmy Abner of Milford, Ohio, age fifteen. His brother was an emergency medical technician, trained in American Red Cross and American Heart Association methods. Timmy was choking and his brother did all the things he was taught by the American Red Cross and the American Heart Association: Hit him on his back, gave mouth-to-mouth resuscitation, put his finger in his throat. This was in the period of several years when the American Red Cross had not accepted the Heimlich Maneuver as yet, and Timmy died while his brother was doing all these things.

In 1976 and '77, an advisor to the American Red Cross was Dr. Archer Gordon, who was also the advisor to the American Heart Association and was on the committee at the National Academy of Sciences that ruled on the treatment of choking. That was the pattern—the same four or five people from 1966 to the present were making the decisions for these organizations. Dr. Gordon's additional qualifications are that he is medical director of an industrial concern and is also, according to an advertising brochure, medical director of a private film company that made films on first aid that show approved American Red Cross and American Heart Association methods.

Dr. Gordon published a paper in which he reported anesthetizing four baboons. He put a piece of meat in their throats, hit them on the back while looking into the throat, and reported that a piece of meat in the throat was loosened. It wasn't expelled but was loosened. His paper also states that he anesthetized six human volunteers and put pieces of meat in their throats but tied a string to the meat so it could be pulled out in an emergency. These were the studies, unpublished at the time, on which the American Red Cross recommended that the first thing to do for choking is to hit a person on the back. Every known published report to that time warned that backslaps were dangerous.

Dr. Harry Gibbons, Director of Health, Salt Lake City and County, objected. He participated at the American Red Cross meeting where backslaps were made the first treatment for choking. He objected to the fact that what had been written up and published by the American Red Cross was not the consensus of the meeting. Dr. Gibbons published an article, "The Biopolitics of Choking," in *The Utah State Medical Journal*, in 1980, in which he told that he was never invited again to one of the American Red Cross, National Academy of Sciences, or American Heart Association meetings on choking—even though he was the first one to institute an anti-choking program in this country and virtually wiped out choking as a cause of death in his area. He was just never invited back.

Another Red Cross/Heart Association/National Academy of Sciences advisor, Dr. Charles Guildner, did a study on humans similar to Gordon's study. His observation was: "The technique of delivering a sharp blow between the shoulder blades was also applied several times. This procedure was so ineffective in creating air flow or increased pressure within the chest, it was abandoned." After he submitted this paper to the *Annals of Emergency Medicine* (then *JACEP*), the American Red Cross came out and said you should slap someone four times on the back before doing the Heimlich Maneuver.

Despite the results of his own study, his conclusions in that same paper, published in 1976, state that when complete airway obstruction is recognized, the following sequence should be applied with the victim sitting or standing: (1) backblows, four in rapid succession; then, if ineffective (2) the abdominal thrust (the Red Cross name for the Heimlich Maneuver) or the chest thrust.

The figure "four" is kind of interesting. I was at the meeting at the American Red Cross where they discussed how many backblows should be used first. Someone said, how about twelve, and someone else said no, they'd be dead by that time. Another person said, how about two? They said no, it'll look like we're not doing anything, and they agreed on four. Recently, in the medical journal *Pediatrics* was a letter to the editor from the Chairman of the American Heart Association Emergency Cardiac Care Committee. He had been questioned on why four backblows are recommended. He answered that four is an easy number to remember.

Since there wasn't much evidence for the backblows that were being recommended, the American Heart Association undertook to circularize their people and find out if they had any experiences with choking. They got a few hundred replies which were supposedly analyzed; however, with the analysis sent out to various people was a letter from the American Heart Association head of data processing to the committee at the Heart Association. The letter said, "These data must be used with extreme care; there is no standard methodology or controls," and it goes on to say how relatively useless this entire study was.

They didn't know in what order different treatments for choking were used. What they did is say that anyone who was saved using a combination of backslaps, fingers in the mouth, or the Heimlich Maneuver—in whatever order—was saved by all three. As a result, with 200 and some odd cases reported, they have 500 saves.

One child caused a great deal of problems for the American Red Cross and Heart Association. Gary Daniels, age fourteen, was in school. He started choking on a peanut butter sandwich but was still breathing. His teacher hit him on the back twice, and drove the object down. He stopped breathing and fell unconscious. By the time they did the Heimlich Maneuver on him and it expelled the bread from his throat, he was brain damaged. At the time the suit against the school came to trial, he had been in a coma three years. As a result, the school awarded Gary's family a settlement of $352,000. The Red Cross, faced with some publicity on this, sent a Telex to its managers and selected chapters, and here's how they described the incident: "In an incident June 11, 1975, in a Harrisburg, Pennsylvania, school, in which a youthful, exceptional student was involved in a choking accident, the victim received first aid at school. After release from the hospital July 8, 1975 (one month later), he is presently at home." Nothing is stated about the fact that he came home in a coma, nothing is stated about the fact that he is still in a coma, nothing is stated about the fact that in the court testimony, which they claim to have read, a teacher stated that she followed the American Red Cross instructions in treating his choking episode. The American Red Cross also said that Dr. Heimlich's deposition was not offered or accepted in evidence by the court, which is true. I had left the country and had given a deposition under oath before both attorneys. For a week the trial went on with doctors' and others' testimony, including that of the Red Cross. At the end of the week, when my testimony was about to be read, the school settled for $352,000. The American Red Cross telex says: "The case was settled on October 12, 1978, following a court order approving a petition for compromise settlement and distribution of settlement proceeds." The American Red Cross also said it was settled without court-established negligence, omitting the fact that there was a $352,000 settlement, the largest in the history of the court in Harrisburg.

DROWNING

Within a year after the Heimlich Maneuver was introduced, we began receiving reports from first aiders and eventually from a doctor who was Chief Fire Surgeon of Washington, DC, and an advisor to the American Red Cross on water safety, of drowning victims being given mouth-to-mouth resuscitation without success. Off the top of their heads, they did the Heimlich Maneuver in the lying-down position. All said the same thing: "The water gushed out and the person recovered." So, I investigated, looking up the literature on drowning.

From the Middle Ages, rolling a person over a barrel, face down, was the successful treatment for drowning. In Germany, in the 17th and 18th centuries, along the canals, they would drape a drowning person face down over the back of a horse and trot the horse. In the early 1900s came the Schaefer prone pressure method: With a person lying facedown, the rescuer pressed on the lower ribs, saying, "Out goes the bad air, in comes the good air." What they were doing in each instance was pushing up on the diaphragm. The horse and the barrel, were doing the Heimlich Maneuver, and so was the Schaefer procedure. The American Red Cross adopted the Schaefer method in 1925, after it had been established for quite a few years, and they taught it until the 1960s.

In 1960, mouth-to-mouth resuscitation came along. The same group of American Red Cross doctors we were talking about before appreciated the fact that mouth-to-mouth resuscitation was indeed the best method of getting air into the lungs, so they said it must be used for drowning as well as for heart attacks and electrocution.

Their instructions, when the Schaefer prone pressure method was used, had been to not waste time by trying to tilt a person to get water out of the lungs, because it won't come out; artificial respiration would in any case squeeze the water out of the lungs. From 1960 to today, the instructions say not to tilt anyone to get water out of the lungs as it will do no good, so proceed immediately with artificial respiration. With mouth-to-mouth artificial respiration, however, the water was not squeezed out of the lungs. Since 1960 the death rate from drowning has constantly increased in this country.

Here is an experiment: You know it takes millions of dollars to do an experiment today; this one costs $2.50. Go to the local bar and order a scotch and soda. You know from childhood that if you dip the straw into fluid and put your finger over it, the fluid will be held in the straw because atmospheric pressure holds it in place. That's why in tilting a drowning victim, water won't come out of the lungs. If you squeeze a plastic straw, though, the water will come out and the straw will pop open filled with air. The Schaefer prone pressure method did indeed squeeze the water out of the lungs, as does the lying-down position for the Heimlich Maneuver. There is no question that you must get the water out of the lungs before you can get air in. Mouth-to-mouth resuscitation has been unsuccessful because the water has not been expelled from the lungs.

On advising the American Red Cross and the American Heart Association of these facts, the first response was that, when you press on the abdomen to do the Heimlich Maneuver, you're going to squeeze up stomach contents and the victim will aspirate it. In a published article *(Annals of Emergency Medicine,* 10: 476, 1981), I pointed out that the victim is not going to aspirate because the reason you treat drowning victims is they are not breathing and they can't aspirate until they breathe. If you do the Heimlich Maneuver to get water out of the lungs and they start breathing, they may aspirate a little, although that has never occurred, but if you don't do the Maneuver, they're going to die. The Red Cross still is not acting on this important, scientifically proven method of saving the life of a drowning person.

RESUSCITATION

Cardiopulmonary resuscitation is being taught to millions of people in this country. They have been told to press on the chest. Recently, however, articles have raised the question, "Does CPR do more harm than good?"

Many of those being saved with CPR have brain damage. A study in 1981 from Johns Hopkins University, published in *JAMA* (246:351), showed that when you press on the chest, as in CPR, you are *not,* as was thought, squeezing the heart between the breastbone (sternum) and the vertebral column. You cannot do that without crushing the chest. They found that what happens with CPR is that the pressure within the chest is increased. This results in higher pressure in the blood vessels in the chest than outside in the neck and brain; therefore, blood flows to the brain and the rest of the body. They noted that pressing on the chest is relatively ineffective since the resulting intrathoracic pressure is dissipated because it causes the diaphragm to descend. The Johns Hopkins researchers, therefore, recommended putting an inflated pillow against the abdomen and tying it around the body with a binder which pushes the diaphragm upward, in effect performing a Heimlich Maneuver. The pressure inside the chest is thereby increased.

Subsequently, at Purdue University, it was proved that the Heimlich Maneuver, pushing up on the diaphragm in the lying-down position, produces maximum intrathoracic pressure and therefore much higher blood flow through the carotid blood vessels to the head and through the aorta to the rest of the body. A study is going on at Purdue and the University of Southern Alabama using this method.

In addition, there are multitudinous reports of crushed chests and deaths due to CPR, one from the Mayo Clinic, of CPR done in their hospital by their doctors in the operating room. Death was frequently due to the crushed chest rather than to heart disease. Hundreds of such cases have been reported (*Pediatrics,* 70:120, 1982).

The facts I've spoken about today are not solely my studies but are published from leading institutions. We must conclude that methods taught by the American Heart Association and the American Red Cross are causing deaths. The reports are published; therefore, those agencies must be aware of this. The American Red Cross and American Heart Association instructions for treatment of a choking victim state that if a person is coughing or breathing or making a sound, don't do anything. Why? Because they know that if the victim's airway is partially obstructed, and you hit the person on the back, the object will wedge tighter. What they don't say is that the Heimlich Maneuver always causes a flow of air away from the lungs, toward the mouth, and therefore, that danger does not exist.

The American Red Cross and American Heart Association have modified their position, however, as follows. Originally they advised to hit the back; then, not to hit the back unless it's a last resort because it's dangerous; Subsequently, they recommended hitting the back first before doing the Heimlich Maneuver. The American Red Cross and American Heart Association position now is that you can hit the back before or after doing the Heimlich Maneuver. Can you see any sense with the mother of a choking child who may die in four minutes worrying which step to do first and how?

This year, the AMA Emergency Medical Services Committee staff met privately with Dr. Archer Gordon and decided the AMA would adopt the American Heart Association's stand. Now the AMA says if someone is choking you can hit the victim on the back either before or after doing the Heimlich Maneuver. It's funny, and it's sad.

QUESTION AND ANSWER PERIOD

Q: I'm a naturopath. The American Red Cross says that if you're going to do CPR then there's a ratio of 15 compressions to two ventilations, if you're by yourself or five compressions to one ventilation if you are with another colleague. What is the ratio that you would suggest; do you do 15 compressions to two ventilations?

Dr. Heimlich: I don't know that the American Red Cross ratio has

A person choking on food will die in 4 minutes - you can save a life using the HEIMLICH MANEUVER*

Food-choking is caused by a piece of food lodging in the throat creating a blockage of the airway, making it impossible for the victim to breathe or speak. The victim will die of strangulation in four minutes if you do not act to save him.

Using the Heimlich Maneuver* (described in the accompanying diagrams), you exert pressure that forces the diaphragm upward, compresses the air in the lungs, and expels the object blocking the breathing passage.

The victim should see a physician immediately after the rescue. Performing the Maneuver* could result in injury to the victim. However, he will survive only if his airway is quickly cleared.

If no help is at hand, victims should attempt to perform the Heimlich Maneuver* on themselves by pressing their own fist upward into the abdomen as described.

WHAT TO LOOK FOR

The victim of food-choking:

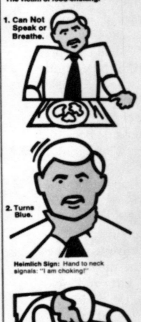

1. **Can Not Speak or Breathe.**

2. **Turns Blue.**

Heimlich Sign: Hand to neck signals: "I am choking!"

3. **Collapses.**

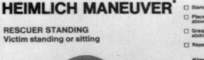

HEIMLICH MANEUVER*

RESCUER STANDING
Victim standing or sitting

☐ Stand behind the victim and wrap your arms around his waist.
☐ Place your fist thumb side against the victim's abdomen, slightly above the navel and below the rib cage.
☐ Grasp your fist with your other hand and press into the victim's abdomen with a quick upward thrust.
☐ Repeat several times if necessary.

When the victim is sitting, the rescuer stands behind the victim's chair and performs the maneuver in the same manner.

OR

RESCUER KNEELING
Victim lying face up

☐ Victim is lying on his back.
☐ Facing victim, kneel astride his hips.
☐ With one of your hands on top of the other, place the heel of your bottom hand on the abdomen slightly above the navel and below the rib cage.
☐ Press into the victim's abdomen with a quick upward thrust.
☐ Repeat several times if necessary

EDUMED, INC.
BOX 52, CINCINNATI, OHIO 45201

© EDUMED, INC. 1976   *T.M. PENDING

any scientific basis. We now know that doing the Heimlich Maneuver is safer and more effective so chances are you might be able to handle it with fewer compressions.

Q: Could you demonstrate it?

Dr. Heimlich: Very simply, all you do is reach around the choking person, feel for the lowest ribs because you don't want to be on the chest, which can cause injury as in CPR. You go below the ribs using the thumb side of your fist. Again, this was scientifically determined. On your fist there's a nice knob on the thumb side. You place the fist below the ribs, almost to the belly button, grasp your fist with your other hand, press inward and upward, and repeat that as many times as necessary. Usually it will be successful on the first or second Maneuver; it depends how experienced the rescuer is. Repeat, however, even up to six times if necessary. People get a little more courage in doing it as time goes on.

Q: Why did you put your hand here on the rib cage and go way below?

Dr. Heimlich: I felt the lower margin of the rib cage because I wanted to stay below it since you don't want to be on the chest. You want to be below it and come inward and upward on the diaphragm, not squeezing but pressing with your fist. Also, the lying-down position as used for drowning victims is very important for treating choking by a young or small person who can't reach around the waist. We had a report of an eight-year-old, as a matter of fact, who threw a man to the ground and saved his life. In the lying-down position, small rescuers can use their weight to do the Maneuver. This was designed so that you sit astride the person's thighs facing him and use your body weight to do the Maneuver. It was also designed so you don't press to either side because there's the spleen on one side and the liver on the other. When you're sitting astride the victim you are going to press in the middle of the upper abdomen. Dr. Archer Gordon convinced the American Red Cross that you should kneel alongside the choking person because then you could do the Maneuver from the side, then run up and give mouth-to-mouth resuscitation as well. That is in the Red Cross printed instructions and posters today. We warned then that if you do the Maneuver from the side you will rupture the liver or the spleen. For three years they taught that, doing it from the side. I don't know how many died, but suddenly, very quietly, three years ago, the Red Cross said to do it in the middle of the abdomen, as I originally described it. Very quietly, so quietly that if you see a Red Cross poster today you will see that the Heimlich

Maneuver is still shown done incorrectly from the side on their newest poster. They have not changed those posters. In fact, those posters are so complicated that you can't tell what to do anyway. They have seventeen pages of instruction in the Red Cross book on treating choking. The thing that makes the Maneuver work is that you can learn it in three minutes.

Q: You're doing the Heimlich Maneuver for cardiac arrest also?

Dr. Heimlich: In the lying-down position.

Q: Just below the rib cage?

Dr. Heimlich: Yes. Because it's the pressure in the chest which causes the flow of blood, as shown by the Johns Hopkins and Purdue studies.

Q: I'm the mother of a lung patient. Now when you say that hitting on the back drives things down farther, well, I'm giving my son a lot of postural drainage treatments which involve hitting him on the back in various positions. Supposedly that should loosen mucus plugs so he will cough them up, or is there something better than that; does that maybe drive some of them down?

Dr. Heimlich: No. If you have him in a postural drainage position that's something totally different. What you're doing is loosening up mucus that is in the base of the lungs and causing him to cough it up. That's quite different from an object that's impacted in the throat.

Q: Some mucus, though, is in the bronchial tubes and down the throat. Wouldn't that make it go back down into the lungs?

Dr. Heimlich: You have to cough that up. About 30 years ago a Chicago anesthesiologist at Cook County Hospital wrote a very excellent paper on mouth-to-mouth resuscitation, but almost all his subjects were adults—I think there were about three toddlers in the group that he had worked on, and only one of those was under one year of age. The Red Cross started recommending mouth-to-mouth respiration, which is an excellent way to move air, provided there's no obstruction, for all ages. Dr. Mendelsohn and I know of one case where a newborn infant who was resuscitated in the hospital by mouth-to-mouth respiration suffered a bilateral pneumothorax and died. So, for a 200-pound practitioner or nurse to try to blow up a six-pound baby's lungs without sufficient caution is a very dangerous procedure. There was a recent article in the *Israeli Medical Journal* of an adult in whom bilateral pneumothorax was caused by mouth-to-mouth respiration. And, of course, in many instances, the stomach has been blown up and distended rather than the air going into the lung. But it's still the best way to get air into the lungs, except in a drowning person, where you must first get the water out.

Q: I'm a student who was taught the choking method by the Chicago Heart Association. Based on your lecture here today, it would be OK then to leave out the four blows before we do the Heimlich Maneuver, is that correct?

Dr. Heimlich: It is not only OK, it is lifesaving. It's interesting that in Illinois when they were about to pass a law saying that the Heimlich Maneuver must be posted in restaurants (this happened in several other states, too), the Red Cross and Heart Association representatives met with people in the health department and said, "Here, we'll let you use our posters for nothing," not telling them there was any controversy. Their poster, with the four backblows, is now posted in Illinois. The Utah State Health Department, on the other hand, examined the scientific evidence, and passed a regulation that no one can be taught to hit on the back to save a choking victim; just the Heimlich Maneuver is taught. Florida passed a law to that effect, and New York City also did a thorough investigation and determined that you must not hit people on the back. Just from posting the Heimlich Maneuver in restaurants, New York City had a 29 percent decline in choking deaths in the first year. Arizona had a 45 percent decline in choking deaths when the Maneuver was taught for two years. There is no known decline in choking deaths published from states teaching backslaps.

Q: I didn't think I was going to be making a comment, but I'm obliged to make a comment because I feel very strongly about what you've been saying here today. I'm an emergency room physician and each time that I apply for privileges or employment as an emergency room physician, I have to go through an elaborate defense of my mechanisms of conducting cardiopulmonary resuscitation because I do not use the backblow method. To this very day, that method is still taught not only by CPR but the ACLS (the Advanced Cardiac Life Support), a program that's designed for physicians. So people should be aware that the majority of physicians who are working emergency rooms are probably using the ACLS system.

You have made a nice contribution and, seeking to find some kind thing to say, the words of a scripture come to my mind: "Well done, good and faithful servant."

Dr. Heimlich: Thank you very much.

Q: Doctor, my name is Arlene Ginata and I wasn't quite sure—are you saying that, in CPR, the Heimlich Maneuver replaces the compressions?

Dr. Heimlich: It should.

Q: At the same rate?

Dr. Heimlich: Yes.

Q: Dr. Heimlich, is the Red Cross opposed to the Heimlich Maneuver? I don't quite understand it: Is it just personal antagonism or stupidity or being stuck in the past? What is the actual reason for it?

Dr. Heimlich: Well, first of all, let's understand something. There is no question about the Heimlich Maneuver. The Red Cross teaches the Heimlich Maneuver, the Heart Association teaches it, the AMA teaches it, everyone teaches the Heimlich Maneuver, public health agencies worldwide. So, the question really is: Why do they teach this other stuff with it that has been disproven for so long? One answer is that this same group of people who are teaching backslaps was responsible in 1966 and 1973 for the present standards of those organizations, and they simply made a mistake. In fact, since 1933, they had made the mistake of using backslaps in the treatment of choking and people said to them, after the Heimlich Maneuver came out, why are you doing this? Here is this medical literature of more than 130 years in which all the experts showed evidence to the contrary. Perhaps the continuation of backslaps is partly fear of legal action against the organizations that taught them for many years. I don't know, perhaps because of pride or whatever they hung on to the backslaps. They did it, and they have no acceptable scientific evidence for it. It's tragic, again for me particularly, because my desk is a clearing house for reports of the deaths that occur.

Q: Dr. Heimlich, I have to tell you that a few years ago in Illinois, every physician who had not received CPR training in medical school had to get that kind of training. So I went to the seven sessions or whatever it was and watched how they were teaching everybody, and they had clearly taught us about the backslaps. And somebody in the class asked about the Heimlich Maneuver. The class instructor said, "What we're teaching you *is* the Heimlich Maneuver." And this person tried to argue with the teacher and it turned into a kind of donnybrook. So I was happy to find out that right after I finished taking the course, the state dropped it as a requirement for medical licensure.

But I would like to ask you something. It would be nice to know why the American Red Cross and the Heart Association behave that way, but I'm not particularly interested in their motives. What I am interested in is again, as John McKnight said this morning, what can citizens do? Wouldn't the proper answer be the next time the American Red Cross comes to solicit, I should tell them I'm sending my money to the Heimlich Institute? At least is seems to me that's one possibility.

Dr. Heimlich: I won't argue with that.

Q: The other question I'd like to ask you is either a generic or possibly an extrapolation of what you said. I learned a long time ago when I was in the armed forces in the Second World War not to trust the Red Cross because at the time they were still segregating blood, and even today I don't trust the Red Cross exceedingly. So what I'd like to ask you is, if the Red Cross and the American Heart Association cannot get it straight on the Heimlich Maneuver, can they get it right on anything else?

Dr. Heimlich: You can go through many things they do, such as selling coffee to the troops during the war. The Salvation Army, which is a wonderful organization, gave it away for nothing. You have to attend their policy-making meetings to understand what goes on, and you have to look into what was done.

I went to the National Academy of Sciences (NAS) meeting to which Dr. Gibbons was not invited. The same Red Cross group was there on the choking panel, plus one or two others. There were also about 50 or 60 invited doctors and scientists who just wanted to sit there and listen to the discussion, but the chairman said they were not going to allow any outsiders in this meeting. I said, "Wait a minute, there's a sunshine law." He said, "We don't have to obey the sunshine law; we've gone through that legally."

(In case you think this NAS thing is an isolated incident, there's a good report about it by Philip Boffey of the Ralph Nader Organization. He spent two years with the NAS and reports that the way decisions come out depends on who sponsors an NAS study [*Science*, May 1973, p. 574].)

We went into another private session, and from 7 to 11 o'clock at night, discussed something totally unrelated to choking. We got into choking between 11 o'clock and 12 o'clock at night, when everyone wanted to quit. To end it, I simply made a motion that the Heimlich Maneuver is the best method for treating choking and it passed—six of them passed it, two voted against it. The next morning, when the report was made by the chairman to the entire group there, he said the meeting on choking went on until midnight and no conclusions had been reached. I have this documented, by the way, in the minutes. Someone also said, "Good, now we can keep the Red Cross booklet."

I am talking about the bureaucracy up on the top. There are wonderful people in both the Red Cross and the Heart Association, really dedicated people. Many of the instructors, as a matter of fact, have written to me and said that they have to teach what they're told so that people can get their cards, but then the teachers tell them to forget about the backslaps. There are wonderful people in the organizations, volunteering and working, but the methods are determined by a small group.

Q: In the early stages of CPR development, can you explain to me why, before the compression, they used the brutal act of slapping with the butt of the fist, pounding the victim or the patient, and then starting the compression? And why was it then suddenly deleted without explanation?

Dr. Heimlich: The precordial thump. I read about that in a paper, showing the injuries from compressing the chest. That also happened in first-aid classes. Chests were crushed, and that's why they now use mannequins. There's a marvelous paper by one of the Red Cross people which showed that, in normal people or in people who had fainted, the precordial thump caused ventricular asystole and the person died from a bruised heart. When I wrote this up, there was a letter to the editor from the Heart Association representative, in which he said this was never the case, that they never had injuries from the precordial thump; they just gave it up. In reply, I simply quoted the paper, which was from their own organization, showing that they did give it up for that reason. I don't know how many people died, but we have innumerable reports in the literature about that.

Q: A very quick question: Are there any dangers of lacerating the spleen or liver with the xiphoid process? You mentioned the straightforward compression versus from the side, and when I took CPR, they made a very big deal about making sure that we were not compressing around the xiphoid process. I was just wondering with the Heimlich Maneuver, and also with CPR, what are the risks in terms of that kind of laceration?

Dr. Heimlich: Well, what I've shown you is that you go below the rib cage in the middle and you don't squeeze, you press upward under the diaphragm; so, we don't know of any such cases. There was a very good study done by Dr. Trevor Hughes, University of North Carolina. He contacted 10 or 20 forensic pathologists and the editors of pathology journals and asked if they had ever had knowledge of an injury from the Heimlich Maneuver and none of them had. There will be injuries, let's not mistake it, particularly by those who do it wrong. The Red Cross and Heart Association teaches, again because of the Guildner paper (*JACEP*, 5: 675, 1976), that you can either do the Maneuver on the abdomen as I've shown you or on the chest.

POSTSCRIPT

As far as we can tell, as a direct result of the publicity generated by Dr. Heimlich's lecture at the *Dissent in Medicine* meeting, the American Heart Association and the American Red Cross reversed their positions of the past ten years. At the 1985 National Conference on Standards and Guidelines for Cardiopulmonary Resuscitation and Emergency Cardiac Care in Dallas on July 11, 12, and 13—a conference sponsored principally by the American Heart Association, with the American Red Cross, the American College of Cardiology, and the National Heart, Lung and Blood Institute—these major first-aid groups rejected the backslaps and adopted the Heimlich Maneuver as the *only* approved emergency treatment for choking victims.

Before this decision, the American Red Cross had used the somewhat confusing and misleading term "abdominal thrusts" to refer to the Heimlich Manuever. Following the Dallas meeting, however, Dr. Heimlich wrote to the president of the American Red Cross, saying: "Now that back blows have been removed from the treatment of foreign body obstruction, I have no objection to the American Red Cross using the name 'Heimlich Maneuver.' " The conference's decision will require significant rewriting of first-aid manuals and literature and changes in first-aid training.

In the *Los Angeles Times*, July 23, 1985, Dr. Lewellys Barker, Red

Cross CPR director, is quoted as saying that the Red Cross does not believe backblows are unsafe. "We don't think there is tremendous public health risk in using what people have been taught in the past (backblows)." That statement subjects millions of people trained by the Red Cross for the past ten years to the dangers of backblows. They are not being advised of the extensive scientific evidence presented at the Red Cross/Heart Association meeting that proved that backblows are ineffective for choking victims and cause deaths.

The Red Cross also eliminated "chest thrusts" as a first-aid treatment for choking, a method they taught for ten years. Dr. Heimlich had warned repeatedly of the crushed chests and other injuries caused by such chest compressions.

Also at the Dallas conference, the Heimlich Maneuver was, for the first time, officially approved as an emergency treatment for drowning victims. At a panel, Dr. Jerome H. Modell of the University of Florida College of Medicine said he would recommend that the Heimlich Maneuver be used after a near-drowning victim does not respond to mouth-to-mouth resuscitation. Dr. Heimlich agreed with the recommendation—with the qualification that those who believe it would be more effective would be permitted to use the Maneuver first.

Dr. Heimlich had presented numerous reports of drowning victims having been saved by the Heimlich Maneuver after mouth-to-mouth resuscitation had failed to revive the victim. The reason is that the Heimlich Maneuver expels water from the lungs and *you must get the water out of the lungs before you can get air in.* The proper method for saving a drowning victim, Dr. Heimlich emphasized, is to do Heimlich Maneuver in the lying-down position, as the first step, to get water out of the lungs; when water no longer flows from the mouth, should the victim not recover, proceed with mouth-to-mouth resuscitation. In all reported cases, however, all victims recovered with the Heimlich Maneuver alone. *(RSM)*

CORRUPTION IN AMERICAN MEDICINE

Alan S. Levin, M.D.

INTRODUCTION OF THE SPEAKER

Professor Sorey: Our next speaker will be Dr. Alan Scott Levin, who currently is Adjunct Associate Professor of Immunology and Dermatology at the University of California, San Francisco, School of Medicine. Prior to this, he was Director of the Laboratory of Immunology, University of California, and Kaiser Foundation Research Institute, San Francisco, and Director of the Division of Immunology, Western Laboratories in Oakland, California.

Dr. Levin completed medical school at the University of Illinois, Chicago Medical Center, and trained at Children's Hospital Medical Center in Boston. He is the recipient of fellowships, grants, and awards from Harvard Medical School, United States Public Service, and the American Cancer Society. Among the many professional organizations with which he is affiliated, Dr. Levin is a Certified Diplomate of the American Boards of Allergy and Immunology and Pathology. He is a Fellow of the American College of Emergency Physicians, the College of American Pathologists, and the American Society of Clinical Pathologists. He has coauthored two books, *A Consumer Guide for the Chemically Sensitive* (1982) and *Type I/Type II Allergy Relief System* (1983).

LECTURE*

Dr. Levin: Mr. and Mrs. J are a couple. Mr. J is an attorney in San Francisco and Mrs. J is a Certified Public Accountant with a thriving practice in Santa Clara. They have three children, the oldest six, the youngest eleven months. Since they are not inexperienced, hysterical parents they were not terribly troubled with their youngest child's chronic, intermittent diarrhea until it continued for over six months. Being well-educated people, they sought the best pediatrician in the area. They were pleased when they could have their child seen by Dr. X, a senior professor at Stanford University. Dr. X was an experienced, well-respected physician in his early fifties who spoke with authority. He took the history and performed a physical on the child. He then said to Mrs. J, "Now, honey, Jimmy is a fine boy. His diarrhea is functional. It bothers you more than it does him. All he needs is a little Kaopectate; you need a little Valium." Mrs. J resented the condescending nature of the professor, but more so, she did not feel comfortable with his diagnosis. Through a friend she found an alternative-care physician, one who is dedicated to the study of diseases caused by foods and environmental agents as well as bacteria and viruses. This physician prescribes fewer drugs than the ordinary doctor and often implements dietary and environmental changes in lieu of drugs for various complaints. The alternative-care physician said, "Mrs. J, your son may be allergic to cow's milk. Let's try a simple elimination diet for a few weeks and see what happens." Sure enough, two days after discontinuing milk, little Jimmy's stools became normal. Mrs. J was furious. She came to me and shouted, "Doesn't Dr. X at Stanford University know about milk allergy?" My answer was, "I can think of only two reasons that Dr. X may not have considered milk allergy. Either he is ignorant of the copious amount of literature published on the subject, or he has a vested interest in the routine distribution of large amounts of drugs."

Health care in the United States has become a megabillion-dollar business. It is responsible for over 12 percent of the gross national product. Revenues from the health industry, which currently exceed $360 billion a year, are second only to those of the defense industry. True profits are much higher. It is not difficult, then, to see why this industry is so appealing to corporate investors. Many industrialists determined to

---

*Dr. Levin requested that this paper be included in place of the ad hoc remarks he made at the *Dissent in Medicine* meeting. Accordingly, the questions and answers that followed his talk are not included here.

profit from health-care products have encountered one major obstacle: Practicing physicians remain the primary distributors of health care products. Physicians, who have traditionally existed as independent entrepreneurs do not fit easily into the corporate mind-set. If corporations did not have control over their distributors (the physicians) they would not be able to guarantee profits to their stockholders. With the present premarketing cost of research and development for each new drug exceeding $7 million, a corporation may risk investing millions of dollars in the development of a drug which may subsequently be deemed ineffective. Although this may be good medicine, it is unquestionably bad business. Thus, we need not wonder why senior executives of major health care-oriented corporations have decided to woo physicians into their camps.

Pharmaceutical companies have curried the favor of practicing physicians for many years. During the early 1960s, in reaction to the thalidomide scare (a sedative used during pregnancy which ultimately caused severe birth defects), the U.S. government markedly increased federal drug regulations. Prior to this period, the FDA regulated the toxicity of products released to the general public. After the thalidomide episode, the FDA's mandate was expanded to regulate the efficacy of drugs as well. These changes dramatically increased the cost of development of drugs. As the cost of development and marketing of pharmaceuticals increased, the drug companies efforts to attract the allegiance of practicing physicians intensified.

Not only did drug company operation costs increase markedly, but the rewards of the marketplace rose tremendously. An increase in federal funding for health-care programs, coupled with the general public's heightened awareness of their own health, caused drug industry revenues to soar into the 20 to 30 billion-dollar market it is today. The increase in revenues brought competition which led to a nationwide increase in drug advertising. Advertisements in medical journals and public magazines were popularized by carefully controlled news releases associated with "medical breakthroughs."

These advertising efforts, which began with gifts to practicing doctors and medical students, have become a massive campaign to mold the attitudes, thoughts, and policies of practicing physicians. Drug companies hire detail men to visit physicians' offices and to distribute drug samples. They describe the indications for these drugs and attempt to persuade physicians to use their products. Like any other salesman, they denigrate the products of their competitors while glossing over the shortcomings of their own. Detail men have no formal medical or pharmacological training and are not regulated by any state or federal agencies. Despite their lack of training, these salesmen have been very effective. Their sales campaigns have been so successful within the United States that the average physician today has virtually been trained by the drug detail man. This practice has led to widespread overuse of drugs by both physicians in their everyday practice and the lay public. A recent study has shown that one out of three hospitalizations today occurs as a direct result of the mismanagement of prescription and over-the-counter drugs. With the exception of heroin and cocaine, 85 percent of all drugs currently abused in the streets are manufactured by "ethical" drug companies. More than 85 percent of a certain tranquilizer manufactured today is used illegally! Gross sales forecasts from these "ethical" drug companies deliberately include profits made from illicit sales to drug peddlers.

The drug industry woos young medical students by offering them gifts, free trips to "conferences," and free "educational material." Young physicians are offered research grants by drug companies. Medical schools are given large sums of money for clinical trials and basic pharmaceutical research. Drug companies regularly host lavish dinner and cocktail parties for groups of physicians. They provide funding for the establishment of hospital buildings, medical school buildings, and "independent" research institutes.

The pharmaceutical industry has purposefully moved to develop an enormous amount of influence within medical teaching institutions. This move was greatly facilitated by several factors. The first was the economic recession, which caused a marked constriction in federal funding for research programs. Academic scientists lacked funding for pet research projects. The second was the tremendous interest that academic scientists held in biotechnology, the stock market, and the possibility of becoming millionaires overnight. The third is the fact that academic physicians tend to lack real clinical experience. In the university, the physician is an expert in esoteric disease, end-stage disease, and animal models of human disease. He or she has little or no experience with the day-to-day needs of the chronically ill patient or the patient with very early symptoms of serious illness. As the academic physician does not depend upon the good will of the patient for his or her livelihood, the patient's well-being becomes of minor consideration to him or her. All of these factors make the academic physician a very poor judge of treatment efficacy and a willing pawn of health industrialists.

Pharmaceutical companies, by enlisting the aid of influential academic physicans, have gained control of the practice of medicine in the United States. They now set the standards of practice by hiring investigators to perform studies which establish the efficacy of their products or impugn that of their competitors.

Last year, a double-blind controlled study was performed on Inderal, a drug used to prevent sudden death from second heart attacks. Research was halted early on grounds that the overwhelmingly positive results deemed it no longer "ethical" to maintain the placebo control group. The study was published in a prestigious medical journal and pressure was put on the Food and Drug Administration to officially authorize the use of Inderal for this purpose. Much media coverage was afforded this "medical breakthrough" and Inderal is now the standard drug used to prevent sudden death after heart attacks. The real facts relating to this study indicate that the issue had become a question of economic gain and not one of medical ethics. The controlled trial was discontinued too early to allow a scientifically based decision concerning the use of Inderal for this purpose to be made. The statistics were manipulated to make the results look significant. In Switzerland, just prior to this time, a drug called Timolol had undergone extensive double-blind controlled studies and was found to be very effective in preventing sudden death from second heart attacks. The drug had passed all FDA tests and had been approved for use in such patients. Timolol was scheduled to be marketed in the United States within weeks of the announced "medical break-through" on Inderal. It would seem that the manufacturers of Inderal and the academic physicians they hired to perform the study were more interested in maintaining the drug's market share than in the ethics of continuing the trial.

The food industry and the drug industry are closely allied. Drug companies often manufacture the additives used by food processors in the manufacturing of their products. The two industries are regulated by the same federal agency. Kraft Foods, as well as several other large food processing firms, have been bought by drug industry interests. In order to facilitate the development of both industries, the Nutrition Foundation was formed. This is an industry coalition developed to coordinate political lobbying and to support scientific studies for the enhancement of profits. This coalition often sponsors research in very prestigious universities. A prominent Professor of Nutrition at Harvard University recently published a number of studies proving that food additives do not cause hyperactivity in children. He publicly endorses the use of soft drinks, candy, and food additives for children. He advocates that hyperactive children not be treated with elimination diets but with standard drug therapy. Recently, the Nutrition Foundation honored this prominent scientist by funding a laboratory on the Harvard University campus in his name. Standard therapy for hyperactive children involves the use of the drug Ritalin, an amphetamine-like agent. This drug is addicting and can cause psychotic behavior. Ritalin is a favorite form of "speed" in the drug culture. It is one of the most popular street drugs and draws high prices in the illicit drug trafficking trade.

These facts describe only a portion of the problem. Practicing physicians are intimidated into using treatment regimes which they know do not work. One glaring example is cancer chemotherapy. Chemotherapy is lifesaving treatment for leukemias, lymphomas, and several rare carcinomas, but chemotherapy does not work for the majority of cancers. Documented evidence, existing for over a decade, shows that chemotherapy does not eliminate breast, colon, and lung cancers. Documented evidence has shown that studies reporting positive effects of chemotherapy in these tumors have been manipulated to such an extent that the possibility of fraud becomes very real. Most cancer chemotherapy studies consider patients who die of drug toxicity as "unevaluable." These deaths are not factored into the survival statistics. A popular chemotherapy protocol which at present is widely used to treat women with breast cancer originally reported only those results for women whose tumor mass reduced by 60 percent after the first course of treatment. The investigators ignored statistics from women whose tumors did not respond. Despite this glaring omission, the difference in tumor-free survival between the treated and untreated women was only 12 percent. When the original study is carefully evaluated, it becomes obvious that chemotherapy is more likely to *reduce* tumor-free survival! This treatment is now considered the standard treatment for women with breast cancer.

Most physicians agree that chemotherapy is largely ineffective for the majority of cancers. Despite this fact, honest physicians are coerced into using these treatment modalities by special interest groups who have a vested interest in the profits of the drug industry. A physician in California is practicing the standard of care when he treats a colon cancer patient with 5-fluorouracil. He will be rewarded with an insurance reimbursement of 80 to 100 percent. This is true despite the fact that many articles appearing in prestigious medical journals have shown that 5-fluorouracil does not work. The same physician will not be reimbursed for treating the patient with high-dose vitamin C. In fact, he will be in jeopardy of losing his medical license. There is no evidence found in the medical literature supporting the claim that it is dangerous to use nutritional support in the treatment of cancer patients. However, there is voluminous literature supporting the scientific rationale for using this type of treatment.

A similar situation exists in the field of allergy. Lately, the American public has become increasingly interested in nutrition and the impact of foods on their health. This has brought about the recognition of food-associated symptoms in such widely diverse diseases as migraine headaches, asthma, eczema, psychotic behavior, and rheumatoid arthritis.

Food-allergy testing and treatment has been the therapeutic mainstay of more than 1,500 physicians for thousands of patients for more than 10 years. Food-allergy testing and treatment has been the subject of numerous textbooks, American Medical Association-recognized continuing medical education courses, and controlled clinical trials. The American Medical Association and many prestigious medical specialty societies recognize these testing and treatment techniques as safe and effective. This treatment modality, however, has not been generally popular among a small group of academic allergists.

The marked increase in interest has brought the subject of food-allergy testing and treatment to the attention of several special interest groups who have a vested interest in removing these modalities from the market. The incidence of allergic disease has been estimated at close to 30 percent of the total population. Allergy testing and treatment is a multibillion-dollar market. Even a slight change in the way these diseases are treated could result in a bonanza for certain special interest groups. These groups include the food industry, the drug industry, and the allergists who do not perform such testing and treatment. These special interest groups have sponsored a number of scientific investigations which have resulted in the publication of several reports impugning the credibility of these practices. Several of these studies purporting to be unbiased, double-blind, placebo-controlled studies, are clearly unscientific and poorly designed; no credibility could be lent to their conclusions. Despite the obvious scientific and ethical flaws in these studies, the American Academy of Allergy has chosen to use them in their "Official Position Statement on Controversial Practices in Allergy" published in 1981. The American Academy of Allergy and its official publication, *Journal of Allergy and Clinical Immunology*, are heavily funded by the drug industry. Coincident to the publication of this official statement, the Food and Drug Administration has been asked to reevaluate the safety and efficacy of these practices, and insurance companies have been asked not to reimburse patients for such treatment.

The American Academy of Allergy is at present waging a very expensive, well-orchestrated political and economic campaign to persuade the federal government and the insurance industry to limit the medical practices of those physicians who recognize diseases caused by foods and drugs. A combine of academic physicians, with the support of the food industry and the drug industry, are now actively attempting to discredit investigators who have found that food allergy is a major medical problem. They cite several uncontrolled studies to justify their position while ignoring the multitude of scientifically sound studies which acknowledge the prevalence of food allergies. These physicians and their representatives are putting enormous pressure on Food and Drug Administration officials who readily admit that the issues are political and economic, not scientific. The outcome of this battle has yet to be determined.

These are just a few of the facts demonstrating the corruption which exists in the field of medicine as it is today. Your family doctor is no longer free to choose the treatment modality he or she feels is best for you, but must follow the dictates established by physicians whose motives and alliances are such that their decisions may not be in your best interests. You, the taxpayer, the voter, the consumer, can help stop this corruption. You must take control of your own health. If you do not understand why your physician recommends a certain drug or treatment program, ask questions. If your doctor becomes impatient or angry, question his motives and seek medical care elsewhere. Support your doctor when he uses unconventional modes of treatment which you feel have improved your health. If possible, try to cure yourself without the use of drugs. Support your physician if he tells you the truth about the drugs which are considered to be "the standard of practice" in the treatment of a given disease. Recognize that he is risking his livelihood and his personal freedom for your well-being. Write your Congressperson or Senator if your doctor appears to be harassed by the local medical board or the police. Remember that your doctor would rather help you than comply with the edicts of the health industry. With your support, he or she can join the ever increasing number of physicians who have repudiated the tyranny of the health industrial complex.

THE ACCURACY OF MEDICAL TESTING

A Dissenting View—Not to Mention the Terrible Waste of Life, Limb, and Money

Edward R. Pinckney, M.D.

INTRODUCTION OF THE SPEAKER

Dr. Pinckney is a consultant in internal and preventive medicine in Beverly Hills, California. In addition to his M.D. degree, he also has a Master's degree in public health and a law degree. He was formerly an Associate Editor of the *Journal of the American Medical Association* and was an editor of four other medical journals, including one for lawyers. He and his wife Cathey are the authors of 10 medical books; the latest being *The Patient's Guide to Medical Tests* and *Do-It-Yourself Medical Testing*, both published by Facts On File, New York. He was formerly in charge of teaching preventive medicine at Northwestern University Medical School and has been on the faculty of two other medical colleges. He is a Fellow of the American College of Physicians.

*LECTURE**

Dr. Pinckney: Before revealing the shocking lack of accuracy of a great many medical tests, a most peculiar paradox must first be mentioned. And that is: When it comes to being tested, the vast majority of patients—even well people—never seem to care about the true value of a medical test, least of all its usefulness to them personally. What is even worse, all too few people even consider a test's cost—no matter how unjustifiably expensive, nor do they ever give a thought to a test's dangers where, in all too many instances, the risks can be far greater than any benefits.[1, 2]

People who seek out discount stores and generic labels, who spend weeks searching for the very best values, who question every word of a warranty prior to making a purchase, and who are even unwilling to cross the street against a traffic light, will not hesitate to throw caution to the wind when it comes to undergoing medical tests. These people will blindly commit themselves—and those who pay their medical bills—to diagnostic technology that could possibly kill them, bankrupt them, or both.[3] This paradoxical myopic reverence for medical tests should be kept in mind whenever medical testing is discussed, for, in truth, it is the ridiculous worship of—and demand for—medical testing that is the primary cause of the high cost of medical care today, along with the even greater risk to life and limb.

Consider a real-life example. A patient comes to the doctor complaining of occasional pains in and around the stomach area. Depending primarily on the patient's history—the story the patient tries to tell—the doctor attempts to pinpoint the problem. After taking into account age, sex, when the pain first started, whether there have been similar episodes in the past, whether the pain comes and goes, whether it is related to food, and what kinds of food, whether it is related to stress or sleeping, and the answers to a host of other leading questions, the doctor then decides on the most likely diagnosis.

Assume the patient's story seems to focus on the possibility of gallstones. As an integral part of the search for those stones, the most commonly performed medical test is the taking of an X ray of the gallbladder area—after the patient is given some pills to swallow—pills that contain a unique chemical dye. That dye is supposed to concentrate

---

*This lecture was presented via videotape; Dr. Pinckney was not present at the *Dissent in Medicine* conference.

inside the gallbladder and make the stones show up on the X-ray picture. In some instances, the doctor may inject the dye rather than use the pills.

How accurate, and safe, do you imagine that medical test to be? Before answering the accuracy part of that question, you should be made aware that clinical pathologists—doctors who specialize in the mechanics of medical testing—consider any medical test even 80 percent accurate to be a poor test.[4] A good test is accurate 95 percent of the time, while an excellent test must be right at least 97 percent of the time.

Now for the accuracy of the X-ray test routinely used to diagnose gallstones. Articles in medical journals declare that, even when gallstones are actually present in the gallbladder, the accuracy rate for that test averages only from 13 to no more than 30 percent.[5, 6] If the dye is injected rather than swallowed, the accuracy of the test may go to 50 percent, but no higher.[7] With the best of everything going for you—the finest doctor, the most experienced technician and the most modern equipment—you still have less than a 50-50 chance of that test having any value at all. There are articles in the journals that come right out and label these tests for gallstones as "obsolete."[8]

Should you agree to have that test, however, you automatically authorize the expenditure of from several hundred to a thousand dollars or more; much of the cost depends upon who performs the test, where it is done, and how often it has to be repeated—once is rarely enough and three times is considered average. Even if you think you do not pay for this relatively useless test directly, you still do indirectly through your health insurance or your taxes.

And what about the safety of that test? For your money, you not only had the opportunity of being exposed to a large amount of harmful radiation[9] but, it is also a known fact that at least one out of every twenty people who take such a test has some sort of dangerous side effect such as a severe breathing problem, kidney failure, and even mental aberrations.[10] What is even worse, from 200 to 800 patients die every year as a consequence of some related allergic-type reaction from the dye.[11, 12] More recent evidence indicates that these dyes can also cause chromosome damage.[13]

If such a test is so relatively valueless, and so absolutely dangerous, why is it even done? Before answering that question, know that there is a reasonably safe test to detect gallstones that has an accuracy rate of 97 percent. It is called cholecystosonography, and it visualizes gallstones by using ultrasound.[14] In addition, this medical test is not invasive; that means, to perform the test it is not necessary to penetrate the skin or introduce any instrument, needle, catheter, or chemical into any part of the body.[15] But, in spite of its accuracy and relative safety, that particular test usually brings a doctor less than $100. Compare that fee to the several hundreds, or even thousands, of dollars that can come from X-ray testing. Perhaps that will help answer the question of why certain tests are preferred over others by some doctors.[16]

Medical Tests and Money

A Rand Corporation study not only indicated that the use of tests has become excessive, but it also implied that the excessive use was due to the financial incentives inherent in test ordering.[17] And, an article in *The Wall Street Journal* reported: "With patients becoming scarcer, doctors are facing an income squeeze. In-office testing could be a way of generating income."[2, 15-23] Lest you think that money is not a part of the overall testing picture, then know that every day doctors receive an array of articles and advertisements pointedly showing them how to increase their earnings greatly by performing as many tests as possible[24-35]—the appropriateness and safety of such testing is never mentioned. One company that makes office blood-testing equipment tells doctors how they can make an extra $44,000 profit year after year for only a $3,000 initial investment to buy their machine. They need only perform 30 tests a day—or about one or two on each patient they see each day.[36] Another company tells doctors that, if they buy their electrocardiograph machine, that company will furnish free supplies for the first 150 cardiographs.[37, 38] Thus, the machine should pay for itself within a few months and then give a profit of at least $20,000 a year by performing cardiographs on no more than one, or two at the most, patients a day. Should your doctor send your blood out to a commercial laboratory for testing, the charge—to the doctor—for 28 different tests is, in one instance, only $5.50.[39] Of course, money enters into the abuse of medical testing, but—and this is a big but—it is still second to the patient's insatiable desire to undergo all those tests at any cost or risk. Without that unquestioning devotion to being tested, there would be no money factor possible.

This time the complaint is of a burning sensation that seems to start in the pit of the stomach and gets worse as it travels up the chest behind the breastbone; a discomfort most commonly described as "heartburn." It has been reported that almost one out of every ten people suffer from this condition.[40] Doctors call it "gastroesophageal reflux" because its most common cause is the regurgitation of stomach acid—with or without undigested food—back up into the lower portion of the esophagus; the lining of the esophagus is not equipped to withstand the acid's irritation, as the stomach's lining is. Doctors admit—at least among themselves and in medical journals—that the diagnosis of this condition can be made from the patient's history alone in more than half of all cases without one single test.[41, 42] Yet, there are at least 10 different tests now being used routinely to "help" make the diagnosis.[42-45] They include those expensive and dangerous X rays or fluoroscopy (in this instance the patient usually swallows a different chemical called barium, in a sort of milkshake, to outline the upper digestive tract on the X-ray picture or screen). Frequently, the patient is turned upside down while being X-rayed to see if the barium leaks from the stomach back into the esophagus; if it does, it shows that stomach acid could do the same thing. That test is considered only about 33 percent accurate.[46] Some of the other tests for gastroesophageal reflux include: putting an instrument all the way down inside the esophagus to measure the pressure or strength of the muscle ring where the esophagus joins the stomach; wearing an electrode inside the esophagus for 24 hours to see if, and when, acids spew up from the stomach; being given acid to swallow to see if it does, in fact, irritate the esophagus; and it is not unusual for a doctor to look all the way down inside the esophagus and then cut out a piece of the lining to see—under the microscope—whether that tissue looks irritated. Yet, simply noting the pain's relation to mealtime, certain foods, body position, and, of greatest importance, whether the pain is relieved by antacids is usually quite sufficient to make a proper diagnosis. Your health insurance company or Medicare will, without question, reimburse a doctor for ten or more tests should the patient insist on them, or injudiciously submit to them, if the doctor orders or performs them, in spite of the fact that only one of those tests has an accuracy rate greater than 80 percent.

For the one test that has the highest accuracy rating, all a patient need do is swallow a small capsule containing a thin nylon string with one end of the string taped to the cheek. After a few minutes the string is pulled back up—the capsule drops off and is dissolved as is any other medicine capsule—and the acidity, or the pH as it is more commonly called, is noted on that portion of the string that comes in contact with the lower part of the esophagus. If the string shows the presence of acid—especially in relation to any discomfort—there can be little doubt about the diagnosis. This most accurate of all the tests for "heartburn" costs less than $10 and also carries with it the least degree of risk. Undergoing some, or even all, of the other not-too-accurate tests can cost well over $1,000—not to mention all the many associated dangers that include the possibility of hemorrhage, perforation of an existing ulcer, and even the need for surgery to remove a test electrode that breaks off or comes loose. While it is easy to see why some doctors insist on as many tests as the traffic will bear, it is still not easy to see why patients so willingly submit to all that testing without the slightest consideration of worth or danger.

12 Billion Tests Per Year

Few people have any idea of just how many medical tests patients submit to every year. In 1983, more than 12 billion tests were performed in the United States alone. That is more than 33 million tests being done every single day of the year. There are 850 different tests that can be performed on blood alone, only a very few have any bearing on diagnosis or treatment.[47] When all direct and related costs for medical testing are added together—including office visits and hospital charges—the annual bill for medical testing, in 1983, came to about 160 billion dollars, or about half of the entire cost of all medical care.[48, 49]

Understanding a Test's Accuracy

Since accuracy is the theme of this presentation, it is necessary to understand how a test's accuracy is determined; every medical test has an accuracy rating well known to doctors. To put it as simply as possible, the measure of a test's accuracy—sometimes called its predictive value—is arrived at by computing its sensitivity and its specificity. The term *sensitivity* reflects a test's ability to show a positive or abnormal result indicating the presence of the disease being searched for when that disease actually exists in the individual being tested; or, in other words, how often the test is right. A test with 100 percent sensitivity is never wrong—but there are very few of these. As a test's sensitivity rating decreases, the lowered percentage figure denotes how often it will fail to show its expected positive or abnormal result even though the disease being tested for exists in the person being tested. For example, a test with an 80 percent sensitivity rating will fail to diagnose its disease in 20 out of every 100 cases. The other basic determinant of a test's accuracy is called *specificity*. This percentage figure reflects the test's ability to show a negative (normal) result when the disease being tested for does not exist in the individual being tested. The lower the percentage rating of a test's specificity, the greater the chance the test will wrongly show the presence of a disease when that disease does not exist. A test with an 80 percent specificity will give a false-positive result in 20 out of every 100 cases, erroneously implying a healthy individual is suffering from a disease that really does not exist. A test with 100 percent specificity would never give a false-positive result—but there are none of these. When the values of both sensitivity and specificity are combined, they give a reasonable indication of a test's accuracy. A test with a 50 percent accuracy rating will be wrong—and give a false result—once for every two times it is performed.

To be sure, there are a few refinements to this oversimplified explanation, one being *prevalence*. The word considers how common the disease being tested for is in the environment of, or within the population group of, the person being tested; it can have an effect on the test's accuracy rating and, at times, should be taken into account.[50, 51]

Understanding a Test's Significance

While accuracy is the primary factor to be considered when assessing the true value of any medical test, another factor, called *significance,* is equally important—especially when comparing a test's worth to its cost. A highly significant test will show a positive or abnormal result in only a very few different—and not necessarily related—diseases. The most significant test will be positive in only one condition, the particular one being tested for—but there are few, if any, of these. Unfortunately, most medical tests can show a positive (abnormal) result in the presence of many diseases—and they can even give false-positive results as a consequence of physical activity or even the body's position (sitting vs. standing), to mention just a few variables.[52]

The blood test for syphilis is a good example. It can wrongly indicate a patient has syphilis if, at the time of testing, the patient happens to have—or is even recovering from—infectious mononucleosis, pneumonia, certain anemias, or lupus, to mention only a very few, unrelated, conditions. That test can even falsely indicate syphilis in an individual who recently had a smallpox vaccination, or in someone using narcotics.[53] In fact, most of the usual blood tests can show a positive (abnormal) result—indicating from dozens to hundreds of different diseases—in essentially healthy people. The typical enzyme evaluations that are part of most routine blood tests can show a false-positive, or abnormal, result in a healthy person for days simply because the person did nothing more than exercise moderately.[54]

Because so many medical tests are not very significant—and rarely point to any one specific disease—they can cause a great deal of anxiety and even physical problems if their results are accepted at face value or uncritically. If both doctor and patient are not aware of the significance of the medical test being performed, two extremely dangerous outcomes can occur. First, there are all the catastrophic consequences of undergoing more and more tests while trying to find some explanation for the initial false-positive test result. Second, treatment—even surgery—could be implemented for a condition that does not really exist; the latter could be considered the ultimate danger of medical testing.[55, 56]

Although most medical tests—even when performed properly and appropriately—are not too accurate or significant in themselves, two other, directly related facts should also be made known. First, when the commercial laboratories that perform the great majority of tests were evaluated by the Center for Disease Control of the Public Health Service, it was shown that year after year the results of one out of every seven tests were totally in error or, in some way, absolutely useless to apply to the patient being tested.[48, 49, 57] At the present rate of testing, that amounts to more than 4 million erroneous test results being reported back to doctors every day! Second, bad as those statistics are, a California study has revealed that the same tests, when performed in a doctor's office, are even less accurate than when performed in licensed laboratories.[58] As an example of test inaccuracy, an article in the *Journal of the American Medical Association* disclosed that when two diabetes specialists reviewed 334 patients who, as a result of medical tests, were told that they had diabetes, they found that half of those patients were wrongly diagnosed and were being treated for a disease they did not have.[59]

These are just a very few of the known facts illustrating the lack of accuracy of medical tests. While the facts are meant to show how essentially useless a great many tests are, they are also intended to point out the great waste of money that accompanies the uselessness. But, in spite of all these facts—and this knowledge has been around for scores of years—medical tests are still indiscriminately ordered and performed[60-63] not so much as a consequence of scientific principle as they are to satisfy patients' whims. And, even in the face of such supposed progress in diagnostic technology, it might be of surprising interest to know that—while using the very latest tests—doctors still fail to diagnose the probability of less than half of all heart attacks that end in death before the tragedy occurs. This rate of success—or should it better be called a rate of failure?—is no different than it was decades ago. Such a poor diagnostic showing has prompted Dr. George Lundberg, editor of the *Journal of the American Medical Association*, to urge physicians to "stop burying [their] mistakes."[64]

The Dangers of Medical Testing

Perhaps one reason people demand so much medical testing is that not enough stress has been placed on the many dangers directly related to undergoing those tests.[65, 66] Medical journals are replete with horror stories of the unfortunate side effects that regularly accompany test procedures; the illness and deaths from dyes used with X rays are but a small fraction of the misfortunes associated with testing. Hair loss, skin damage, broken and blocked veins, broken and lost catheters, and even electrocution are but a very few examples.

One particular hazard—quite unique to medical testing—while published in a major medical journal, has not been brought to the public's attention. As a preface to this peril, it seems necessary to mention "iatrogenic disease." Most people have heard the term; it means that the real cause of the patient's illness or suffering came directly from the doctor's actions or words—not from a germ, improper living, or genetic defect. More often than not, such an illness is secondary to the doctor's therapy, whether the treatment be a wrong drug, unnecessary surgery, or even improper counsel. But how many people have heard of "Ulysses syndrome"? This appellation was devised by Dr. Mercer Rang of Canada and should be considered a most formidable warning to all patients.[67] Remember the Greek warrior Ulysses? He spent nearly a dozen years searching for trouble and, with each new, unexpected adventure, he also endured greater and greater hazards. When a doctor goes searching for some—any—sort of disease through literally endless medical testing, a patient is very apt to suffer from "Ulysses syndrome"; in this instance, all the physical, mental, and even monetary hazards so disastrously associated with a doctor's "adventurous" medical investigation. Being a victim of "Ulysses syndrome" leaves the patient even more exposed to iatrogenic disease later on when some superfluous or erroneous treatment is applied as a result of all the gratuitous testing.

Every necessary medical test puts you in some degree of jeopardy; every unnecessary medical test—while your doctor plays Ulysses—puts you in that much more needless jeopardy.[68-75] And your vulnerability is not limited to side effects, accidents, and injuries; it has been shown that for every seven tests you have, you are assured of at least one false-positive result with all the subsequent calamities that can come from that fictitious verdict.[48, 49, 67, 75] Should you come up with a normal test result, however, do not assume that means you are free, clear, and healthy. In a 1984 article in *Diagnosis,* the doctor-author told his colleagues that even if their patients have *normal* pulmonary function (lung) test results, they should still never exclude the possibility that those patients could still have lung disease.[76] Now how accurate do you think medical tests really are?

What You Can Do

It is one thing to become aware of the facts concerning the accuracy of medical tests; it is quite another thing to do something about them. If you really are interested in preventing illness, improving and protecting your health, and even saving money on medical bills, several courses of action are open to you. The very first is to become aware of the accuracy—and significance—of any test your doctor orders or plans to perform. At present, the law does not require your doctor to give you this information. All your doctor is required to do is to tell you of any dangers related to a test—no matter how slight—before you give your consent to taking that test. If you cannot remember your doctor informing you of a test's risks the last time you took one, then you should also know that your physical acquiescence to taking that test—such as allowing your blood to be drawn, standing in front of an X-ray machine or simply lying down on a table where the test is to be performed, have been legally interpreted as having automatically given your consent. You supposedly had the opportunity to inquire all about the test and, by submitting your body, you declined that opportunity.

Should you decide to become properly informed prior to taking a test and, after hearing all the evidence, do not feel the odds are sufficiently in your favor to warrant undergoing the test, then your doctor is legally required to tell you all of the possible consequences of *not* going through with the test. This does give you a "second chance" to make up your mind. But, just as a doctor is not required to inform you of how accurate or significant a test is—unless you ask—he is also not obligated to tell you what he plans to do to you on the basis of the test's results—unless you ask. Take advantage of that last query and insist on knowing your doctor's intentions in both circumstances—if the test result is normal and if it turns out abnormal. If both answers are the same, why is the test even needed?[77]

As a rule of thumb, do not automatically agree to undergo any test that is less than 80 percent accurate until that test has been completely justified—the potential benefits versus the known risks—in your particular case. This act alone could save your life—or at least your limb, not to mention your money. If you were properly informed ahead of time, would you really prefer being exposed to X rays and potentially dangerous dyes as opposed to the far more accurate, relatively safe ultrasound test for gallstones? You have the right to know all about medical tests before you have them; if you do not take advantage of that right, then forever hold your dissent against doctors.

The next thing you can do, assuming you have been convinced that far too many, not-too-accurate medical tests are being performed without any scientific justification, is to insist that those who pay your medical bills limit their reimbursement to medical tests that have an accuracy rate of 80 percent or better and whose significance reflects no more than five different diseases (arbitrary, to be sure, but a reasonable place to start).[20, 78] Such a monetary restriction would not mean that less accurate or less significant tests need be abandoned; rather, any not-too-accurate or insignificant test would—if you agree to undergo it—simply be paid for out of your own pocket. Naturally, prior to agreeing to go through with the test and pay for it, you doctor would willingly offer you sufficient information about the test's worth—especially as related to your particular circumstances—as well as all associated perils so as to allow you to come to an informed conclusion on the benefits versus the risks of the test in question. Think how this action alone could protect your health and save you from dangerous as well as useless testing. By having third-party payers of medical bills supporting you in your quest for the test with the most value, you will not be alone in the battle for better and less costly medical care. In the long run, you will not be depriving yourself of the latest diagnostic technology; you will only be depriving yourself of the hazards of "Ulysses syndrome." Most doctors acknowledge—if not openly—that less medical testing will not affect, and especially not lessen, the quality of medical care; the American Society of Internal Medicine has admitted that if patients would participate more in their medical care, especially to the extent of a little direct sharing in the cost of that care, they would end up with far more effective, and ultimately less costly, medicine.[79-81]

The third step you, personally, can take requires your answering a most critical question: How much of a sacrifice are you willing to make to achieve the highest quality medical care? That sacrifice concerns your willingness to give up all the attention medical tests provide. True, you do tend to feel quite important when something is being done to you— be it being stabbed by a needle, photographed by X rays, connected to some Frankenstein-like machine, or by having one or more of your very private orifices invaded and explored. It does not seem out of place to say that an unwillingness to give up your momentary position of prominence—artificial and dangerous though it may be—could well be the explanation of that paradox of the unfathomable love and desire for medical tests, a passion that probably contributes most toward the present-day $160 million annual medical test bill.

Defensive Medicine

No discussion of medical tests would be complete without mention of "defensive medicine." That term describes how doctors perform all sorts of totally uncalled-for, dubious, and dangerous tests, ostensibly to protect themselves against the possibility of losing a malpractice lawsuit should a patient take them to court in the future.[52, 82-87] The American Medical Association admits that at least 75 percent of all doctors regularly practice "defensive medicine."[88] The former president of the Los Angeles County Medical Association goes so far as to say that this superfluous testing unnecessarily raises the cost of medical care by at least $20 billion a year.[88] Doctors, of course, blame lawyers, and our litigious society, for this incongruous situation. And doctors go on to say that they are afraid to appear in front of a jury without records that show they performed every conceivable test that might be brought up by a lawyer as possibly—just possibly—being relevant, no matter how remote, to the patient's complaint. Unfortunately, it has been shown that lawyers can easily convince a jury that a doctor who failed to perform some esoteric test—even if medically unjustified—is guilty of negligence and should be punished. But, if everyone would begin to question the accuracy and significance of all medical tests and the true value of each test in question were made known to jury members, lawyers would no longer be able to impress those juries with not-too-accurate, insignificant, and even irrelevant tests. As a most serendipitous consequence, doctors could not feel they have to order redundant, risky tests solely on a lawyer's behalf, rather than a patient's. Think of the savings in life, limb, and money that would bring.

Being as conservative as possible, if reimbursement were limited to the most accurate and most significant tests, it could reduce overall medical spending by at least $50 billion a year—be it by you, your insurance company, or the government. If legislators could be convinced to make such a policy a part of Medicare, it could possibly reduce the cost of that program by half, leaving more than enough funds in that program to allow full benefits—with far less deductions—for everyone eligible and with no fear of that fund's bankruptcy in the future.

The Stress Electrocardiograph Test

Consider one more commonly performed medical test. Almost everyone is familiar with the stress electrocardiograph test, where the heart's action is recorded during physical exertion—be it on a treadmill, pedaling a bicycle, or walking up and down two steps. That test costs from several hundred to more than a thousand dollars; here the cost seems to depend mostly on the doctor's specialty status or prominence along with the elaborateness of his equipment. At the present time, a health-plan or governmental agency unquestioningly pays the bill for that test; no inquiry is ever made to find out if the test was really required. What is even worse, those who reimburse doctors for that test totally ignore its accuracy rating. While there is an admitted wide discrepancy among doctors as to the test's true value, there are sufficient medical articles that come right out and say that, in essence, the stress electrocardiograph test is less than 40 percent accurate.[90, 91] Dr. George Burch, one of this country's foremost cardiologists and former editor of the *American Heart Journal*, calls it just plain "no good."[92-95] In general, it will only help diagnose unsuspected heart disease—and that is in people who actually do have a heart problem—less than 50 percent of the time. What is even worse, and what brings the accuracy rating of this test down even lower, is that it can show a false-positive result—indicating heart disease exists when it really does not—almost 70 percent of the time.[96, 97] In a governmentally sponsored study of 2,000 people who received the test, the ultimate conclusion was that it is "useless" as a means of predicting heart disease.[98] Should such an essentially inaccurate test be considered a justifiable routine medical expense? If you simply cannot bear to give up that test, then perhaps you will think twice after you learn of one of the many risk factors associated with taking it. For every 10,000 stress tests that are done, at least four people have a heart attack—and one of them dies—while the test is being performed.[99-105] Think about those odds when you want all the attention that particular test brings.

Let Medical Tests Compete

At the present time, there are no governmental regulations or professional standards for medical tests as there are for drugs, automobile tires, and even sports equipment such as tennis balls. A medical test does not have to prove itself accurate, or even useful, to be ordered or performed by a doctor and paid for by whomever is responsible for the bill. Do you believe in competition? Then why not let medical tests compete among themselves with only the most accurate and most significant being eligible for reimbursement? Let a medical test prove itself by merit, since it does not have to by law or regulation, before it is paid for without question.

Only you can stop the waste of money and forestall the numerous inherent dangers related to not-too-accurate medical testing. First, inquire about and question the accuracy, significance, and risk factors of every test. Second, help to see that not-too-accurate medical tests are not reimbursed automatically. Finally, refuse to undergo any test that cannot stand the heat of competition, that does not have an 80 percent or better accuracy rating, or that cannot be justified in your particular case. This last effort, giving up all the attention a test brings you, will be the hardest. Are you willing to make that sacrifice?

Notes

1. V. Royster, "Thinking Things Over," *The Wall Street Journal*, 23 May 1984. In discussing a disagreement between his doctor and the third-party payer of some of his medical bills as to whether several medical tests were needed, Mr. Royster wrote: ". . . maybe I didn't need them, but I got them, and personally I'd rather have had them considering the perilous state of my health at my age."

2. J. McPhee, "A Reporter at Large—Heirs of General Practice," *The New Yorker*, 23 July 1984. A physician in Maine is quoted as saying: "Patients, for their part, never protest charges for tests. The public seems to value tests and procedures to an extent that is not justified by their relative scientific value." Referring to the matter of the money to be made from testing (see notes 17–34), this same doctor says: "The money in medicine these days is in tests and procedures, and this leads to conflicts in interests—to tests that are not necessary."

3. J. Krinsley, "Reimbursement for Medically Unjustified Procedures," *N Engl J Med* 311 (1984): 677. Describes the medically unsound, ethically questionable, and financially burdensome practice of how a patient, without any overt medical problems, can answer an advertisement and have a great many expensive and dangerous tests performed and have his or her insurance plan pay for everything in spite of the fact that the patient's personal physician did not request the tests or feel the patient needed them.

4. R. Gambino, "Editorial Comment: Decision Analysis," *Lab Report for Physicians* 6 (1984): 47–48.

5. C. K. Davis and R. D. Schoffstall, "Correlation of Ultrasonic Gallbladder Studies with Operative Findings," *South Med J* 74 (1981): 781–84.

6. M. Crade, et al., "Surgical and Pathological Correlation of Cholecystosonography and Cholecystography," *Am J Roentgenol* 131 (1978): 227–29.

7. R. E. Miller, "Intravenous Cholangiography: Has It Outlived Its Usefulness?" *JAMA* 244 (1980): 2358.

8. M. W. Goodman, et al., "Is Intravenous Cholangiography Still Useful?" *Gastroenterology* 79 (1980): 642–45.

9. M. F. L. Fleming and V. E. Archer, "Ionizing Radiation: Health Hazards of Medical Uses," *Consultant*, Jan. 1984, pp. 167–84. Considers X rays potentially the most harmful of all nonsurgical diagnostic tests.

10. M. Glickstein, "Reactions to Radiographic Contrast Material," *Diagnosis* 1984, 6(9), pp. 27–37.

11. R. Kellerman, "Reactions to Radiographic Contrast Media," *Am Family Phys* 1981, 23(5): 149–52.

12. *F-T-C Reports* (Chevy Chase, MD 1984), 45(49): 14. Reports that Dr. Paul Greenberger of Northwestern University estimates 550 fatalities from dyes used with X rays each year and from 8–10 percent of all patients will have other allergic-like reactions.

13. F. H. Adams, et al., "Effect of Radiation and Contrast Media on Chromosomes. Preliminary Report," *Radiology*, 124 (1977): 323–26. Also see: *Radiology* 129 (1978): 99–203 and *Pediatrics* 62 (1978): 312–16, for follow-up references.

14. P. M. Krook, et al., "Comparison of Real-Time Cholecystonography and Oral Cholecystography," *Radiology* 135 (1980): 145–48.

15. D. H. Spodick, "Invasive Monitoring Imposes Undetermined Risks," *Cardiovascular Procedures*, Feb./Mar. 1982, p. 10.

16. M. Malach, "How to Stop Medicare Waste—and Improve Care, Too," *Med World News*, 28 Feb. 1983, p. 106. Discusses how reimbursement policies encourage the rush to use expensive technology: "Thus, a cardiologist getting only $50 for a consultation with an angina suspect may keep the visit short and refer automatically for coronary arteriography instead of taking the time to see whether a $500 procedure is warranted.

17. P. M. Danzon, et al., "Factors Affecting Laboratory Test Use and Prices," Rand Corporation (Santa Monica, CA) publication R–2987–HCFA, 1983.

18. P. B. Davis, "Medicare Changes Spur Sales of In-Office Diagnostic Gear," *The Wall Street Journal*, 24 Aug. 1984.

19. H. Nelson, "Are Doctors Hurt by Sick Economy?" *Los Angeles Times*, 27 Aug. 1982. Quotes Tom Paton, president of California Blue Shield: "[Doctors] order more services or tests because they have fewer patients, and it's driving costs up."

20. T. Q. Davis, "Is This **TEST** Really Necessary?" *Med Economics*, 17 Sept. 1984. This article, addressed to physicians, begins: "It's been all too easy for us physicians to order extensive—and unnecessary—tests when third-party carriers were picking up the tab with few questions asked."

21. M. Karpen, "Clinical Lab Arriving in MD's Office," *Med Tribune*, 3 Oct. 1984. Describes how the office laboratory will ". . . be providing a new source of physician income." Also quoted in the article is a product manager for a company that makes the equipment to perform office tests: "The inside lab is a way for physicians to generate additional revenues without seeing more patients and without doing more work."

22. F. Wroblewski, "Office Laboratory Equipment: Should You Consider Automation?" *Postgraduate Med* 1984, 76: 211–18. Doctors are told: "As a rule of thumb, the instrument [blood testing machine] will begin generating a profit when approximately ten tests a week are run."

23. "What's Ahead" column, *Med Economics*, 23 Jan. 1984, p. 284. Describes a survey that revealed 69 percent of doctors have a testing laboratory in their offices for the additional income in-house testing brings.

24. "Survey Report," *Diagnosis*, May 1980: pp. 2–6. This article, on profits from in-office testing, was also reprinted and sent to physicians as part of advertising material by manufacturers of office test equipment.

25. A. Gordon, "The Economics of In-Office Laboratories," *Phys Management*, April 1978, pp. 34–41. Discusses costs vs. profits; how one doctor's office lab grossed $1,200 a week (in 1978), performing 25 or more tests daily.

26. C. D. Benton, "Turning Medical Machines into Money Machines Can Ruin Us," *Med Economics*, 24 July 1978, pp. 63–66. Discusses the use of nonlaboratory office diagnostic and test equipment to enrich doctors.

27. A. M. Epstein, et al., "Office Laboratory Tests: Perceptions of Profitability," *Med Care* 22 (1984): 160–66.

28. A. M. Epstein, et al., "A Comparison of Ambulatory Test Ordering for Hypertensive Patients in the United States and England," *JAMA* 252 (1984): 1723–26. Discusses how the financial incentives and benefits may well contribute to the fact that up to 40 times as many tests are performed on patients with high blood pressure in the United States as on patients in England where financial incentives do not exist.

29. P. E. Griner and R. J. Glaser, "Misuse of Laboratory Tests and Diagnostic Procedures," *N Engl J Med* 307 (1982): 1336–39. Discusses test use to generate income.

30. S. A. Schroeder and J. A. Showstack, "Financial Incentives to Perform Medical Procedures and Laboratory Tests: Illustrative Models of Office Practice," *Med Care* 16 (1978): 289–98.

31. J. D. Snyder and C. Bale, "Will In-Office Lab Testing Remain Profitable?" *Phys Management,* Nov. 1983, pp. 63–72. On the possible impact of governmental regulations, particularly Medicare, on office laboratory income.

32. Advertisement in the *Los Angeles County Medical Association Physician,* 7 March 1983, p. 3. Photo of worried physician holding up empty wallet; part of ad copy reads: "We know where doctors are hurting. . . . Today's doctors are being hit where it hurts the most." Then the ad offers in-office laboratory test equipment and supplies.

33. Advertisement in *N Engl J Med,* 301(22), p. xiv. Photo of in-office laboratory; part of ad copy reads: "By doing lab work in your own office . . . you'll increase profitability." Ad placed by medical supply company that sells laboratory equipment and supplies.

34. Advertisement sent to doctors by direct mail; return mail postcard reads, in part: "Quick-Profits Quick-Chem™ . . . high profits for your practice." For doctor's intitial investment of $995, company will give equipment and $500 worth of supplies.

35. Advertisement sent to doctors by direct mail; descriptive folder included a new one-dollar bill with offer of $1,000 in supplies if doctor purchased the company's Seralyzer® laboratory testing equipment ". . . that not only saves money, but produces *added income* for your office."

36. Part of a packet of information sent to doctors by direct mail on the "Economics of the Mallinckrodt Blood Chemistry System." Several options showed the possible profits for one year and for the next five years, return on investment, etc., depending on the number of tests performed in the office each day or week.

37. Advertisement that appeared in many medical journals (e.g., *Am J Cardiology,* Sept. 1981, p. 29.) Older ads assumed the doctor would charge $20 for a cardiogram and promised a $3,000 potential income on initial investment. More recent ads raised the estimated cardiogram charge to $25 and promised more than enough supplies to cover the cost of the machine. (Today the average price for a cardiogram is $35.)

38. Direct mail advertisement told doctors that if they purchased the company's electrocardiograph stress test system, they would receive free supplies for 100 tests— enough to pay for the whole system.

39. Many commercial laboratories offer physicians extremely low prices (including free

supplies and daily office pick-ups) when they send their patients' specimens for testing. More recently some laboratories have added thyroid testing as part of the overall battery and raised the price for *all* the tests to $11.95. The doctor is free to charge his patients any amount, and for each test individually.

40. D. O. Castell, "Two Better Ways to Measure Acid Reflux," *Patient Care*, 15 Jan. 1979, pp. 74–80.

41. B. A. Bachman, "Gastroesophageal Reflux: Simple Measures Often Suffice," *Postgrad Med*, 1983, 74(5), pp. 133–41.

42. L. Charnas, "Pain from the Stomach: Heartburn and Ulcers," *Consumer Health Reporter*, 1984, 2(8), pp. 3–7.

43. J. E. Richter and D. O. Castell, "Gastroesophageal Reflux: Diagnosis and Medical Treatment," *Int Med for the Specialist*, 1983, 4(1), pp. 64–82.

44. A. L. Rogers and J. Cohen, "Gastroesophageal Reflux Disease," *Current Concepts in Gastroenterology*, May/June 1983, pp. 6–45.

45. S. M. Fink and R. W. McCallum, "The Role of Prolonged Esophageal pH Monitoring in the Diagnosis of Gastroesophageal Reflux," *JAMA* 252 (1984): 1160–64.

46. N. Flomenbaum and L. Goldfrank, "Diagnosing Reflux," *Emergency Med*, 30 June 1984, p. 11.

47. *Annual Report*, 1981, American Hospital Supply Company.

48. E. R. Pinckney, "The Accuracy and Significance of Medical Testing," *Arch Intern Med* 143 (1983): 512–14.

49. E. B. Reilly and E. R. Pinckney, "Medical Testing," *Arch Int Med* 143 (1983): 2014–15.

50. M. D. Burke, "The Importance of Prevalence in the Interpretation of Laboratory Tests," *Intern Med for the Specialist*, 1983, 4(4), pp. 45–59.

51. W. B. Applegate, "Decision Theory for Clinicians: Uses and Misuses of Clinical Tests," *South Med J* 74 (1981): 468–73.

52. C. Pinckney and E. R. Pinckney, *The Patient's Guide to Medical Tests*, 2nd ed. (New York: Facts On File Publications, 1982), pp. xxi–xxiii.

53. Ibid., pp. 250–51.

54. E. Coodley, "The Diagnostic Value of Creatine Phosphokinase Levels," *JAMA* 244 (1980): 831–32.

55. R. J. O'Brien, Personal communication from Centers for Disease Control, Atlanta, 1982. CDC estimates that as many as 42,000 persons may have undergone treatment for tuberculosis over a period of a few months following a false-positive tuberculin test's reaction using one company's test solution.

56. G. W. Brown, "Keeping Personal Values Out of Predictive Values," *Diagnostic Med*, July/Aug. 1984, pp. 39–43.

57. M. Fleisher, "Report on Fecal Occult Blood Testing," *Med Tribune*, 29 June 1983. When Dr. Fleisher, of Memorial Sloan-Kettering Cancer Center, sent out test specimen slides for proficiency testing to laboratories around the country, only 50 percent of the readings (reported results) were correct.

58. R. T. Grayson, "Physician-Office Lab Results Less Accurate than Those of Licensed Labs, study shows," *Med World News*, 9 April 1984.

59. R. W. Turkington and H. K. Weindling, "Insulin Secretion in the Diagnosis of Adult-Onset Diabetes Mellitus," *JAMA* 24 (1978): 833–36.

60. E. T. Wong and T. L. Lincoln, "Ready, Fire! . . . Aim!: An Inquiry into Laboratory Test Ordering," *JAMA* 250 (1983): 2510–13.

61. H. L. Fred and P. Robie, "Gimmicks," *South Med J*, Aug. 1983, p. 953.

62. G. D. Lundberg, "Perseveration of Laboratory Test Ordering: A Syndrome Affecting Clinicians," *JAMA* 249 (1983): 639.

63. J. E. Hardison, "Legs," *Arch Intern Med* 143 (1983): 1014. Dr. Hardison says: "Diagnostic maturity is not having to perform a test to confirm a diagnosis you are sure of from the history and physical examination."

64. M. Herring, "The Jim Fixx Dilemma: Averting Unforseen MI's," *Med Tribune*, 3 Sept. 1984, pp. 1, 9.

65. Comptroller General of the United States, *Report to the Congress: Public Hazards from Unsatisfactory Medical Diagnostic Products* (publication No. MWD-75-52), 1975.

66. B. Schorr, "Medical Device Makers Will Be Required to Tell FDA of Deaths, Serious Injuries," *The Wall Street Journal*, 17 Sept. 1984, p. 1. Until now, reporting of fatalities and serious injuries related to (caused by) diagnostic testing apparatus was voluntary; now that reporting is to be mandatory, it is estimated that about 25,000 such reports will be received each year (ten times what has been usual) and this is expected to include 2,000 deaths and serious injuries annually. At present, the FDA considers 2,000 devices (including X-ray machines) currently being used for diagnosis, surgery, or body implantation risky enough to cause death or serious injury.

67. M. Rang, "The Ulysses Syndrome," *Can Med Assn J* 106 (1972): 122–23.

68. G. D. Lundberg, "Did He Take Something? What Does the Lab Result Mean?" *JAMA* 248 (1982): 83. Dr. Lundberg says: "A laboratory test that is either inaccurate or interpreted inaccurately may be worse than no laboratory test at all."

69. J. W. Williamson, M. Alexander, and G. E. Miller, "Continuing Education and Patient Care Research: Physician Response to Screening Test Results," *JAMA* 201 (1967): 118–22. This article, and the four references that follow, discuss how physicians not only fail to review the results of tests they order but, at times, even fail to follow up on reported abnormal test results.

70. R. S. Wigton, et al., "Chart Reminders in the Diagnosis of Anemia," *JAMA* 245 (1981): 1745–47.

71. K. J. Tomecki, and E. C. Tomecki, "Neglect of Syphilis in Hospitalized Patients," *South Med J* 77 (1984): 1118-20. Another report on how positive, or abnormal, test results are ignored.

72. G. Sandler, "Costs of Unnecessary Tests," *Brit Med J* 2 (1979): 21-24. Routine blood and urine tests were of minimal value, contributing to less than 1 percent of all diagnoses.

73. "Editorial: Evaluation of Laboratory Tests," *Brit Med J*, 20 June 1981, p. 282. Only 2 percent of the biochemistry tests resulted in any action (treatment, change of treatment, change in diagnosis to patients). With X rays, action came about in only 18 percent of patients.

74. L. C. Corman, "Many MDs 'Lack Ability' to Interpret Lab Test Results," *Intern Med News* 1981, 14(3): 45.

75. L. J. Schneiderman, L. DeSalvo, and S. Baylor, "The 'Abnormal' Screening Laboratory Results: Its Effect on Physicians and Patients," *Arch Intern Med* 129 (1972): 88-90.

76. G. M. Tisi, "A Practical Approach to Evaluating Pulmonary Function," *Diagnosis* 1984. 6(8): 71-77.

77. P. E. Dans, "Golden Rule," *JAMA*, 248 (1982): 363. The three rules physicians should go by when (before) ordering medical tests on patients: (1) Order a test as if you would be willing to do all the work yourself; (2) Order a test as if you (the physician) had to pay for it out-of-pocket; (3) Order a test only if you would have it done to you (the physician).

78. "Labor Letter," *The Wall Street Journal*, 18 Sept. 1984, p. 1. Reports that the J. C. Penney Company gives it workers full reimbursement for all laboratory test performed outside a hospital. Many other companies do the same without considering the need—let alone the accuracy—of the test.

79. P. Eastman, "Doctors Highly Skeptical of Proposal to Emulate Foreign Medical Practice," *Phys Financial News*, 15 Aug. 1984, p. 15.

80. C. H. Altschuler, "Use of Laboratory Tests," *Ann Intern Med* 95 (1981): 237. One of Dr. Altschuler's comments: "The increased use of laboratory tests is not accompanied by evidence of better care."

81. A. S. Relman, "The Rand Health Insurance Study: Is Cost Sharing Dangerous to Your Health?" *N Engl J Med* 309 (1983): 1453.

82. M. L. Garg, W. A. Gliebe, and M. B. Elkhatib, "The Extent of Defensive Medicine: Some Empirical Evidence," *Legal Aspects Med Practice*, Feb. 1978, pp. 25-29.

83. E. J. Volpintesta, "Doing What 'Needs' to Be Done," *N Engl J Med* 311 (1984): 266.

84. S. McIlrath, "Cause, Effects of 'Defensive Medicine' Debated," *Amer Med News*, July 1984: 3, 61.

85. O. S. Starr, "Defensive Medicine Driving Up Costs," *Amer Med News*, 8 June 1984, p. 65.

86. F. G. Burke, "X-ray Studies: When and Which to Order,," *Consultant,* Jan. 1977, pp. 229–30.

87. C. R. Hasser, "Editor's Corner—Medical Suits: It's High Time for Rationality," *Patient Care,* 15 Sept. 1984, p. 9–10. "The role of defensive medicine in clinical decision making has progressed from that of bit player to that of star in far too many cases. So much for the sanctity of patient benefit."

88. Fever Chart, "Why Most MDs Practice 'Defensive Medicine,' " *Amer Med News* 20 (28 March 1977): 33.

89. W. S. Weil, "I Don't Care What It Costs, I Want the Best," *Los Angeles County Med Assn Phys,* 4 June 1984, p. 11–13.

90. G. B. Kolata, "Lawsuit Points Up Debate over Exercise Electrocardiograms," *Science* 202 (1978): 1175.

91. J. A. Swets, "Sensitivities and Specificities of Diagnostic Tests," *JAMA* 248 (1982): 549.

92. M. Herring, "Asymptomatic CHD: Probes Get Sharper," *Med Tribune,* 19 Sept. 1984 pp. 1, 13. In the same article, Dr. Paul D. Thompson, of Brown University Program in Medicine, decries "the foolishness of the stress test craze," in view of its past [lack of] accuracy record.

93. H. Blackburn, "The Exercise Electrocardiogram in Diagnosis," *Cardiology* 62 (1977): 190–205. Dr. Blackburn says the exercise (stress) test has taken on a role comparable to that of surgery for nonsurgeons; it has produced a bond welded under stress between physician and patient. The bond, as surgeons know, is not likely to be broken, and must be respected and exploited. To ask nonsurgeons to give up their stress electrocardiograph equipment is the same as asking surgeons to give up their tools.

94. "Carter's Doctor Says He Doubts Effectiveness of Stress Test," *Los Angeles Times,* 28 Sept. 1979. After former President Carter's collapse in a foot race near Camp David, Maryland, Rear Admiral William M. Lukash, the President's personal physician, said he never gave the President the test because its effectiveness is a matter of controversy. He also cited the study by the National Heart, Lung, and Blood Institute that "substantiated the limitations of this test."

95. L. K. Altman, "Mondale's Health Termed Excellent by Physician," *The New York Times,* 30 Sept. 1984. Former Vice President Mondale's personal physician admitted he never performed a stress test on his patient in spite of Mondale's blood pressure problems.

96. "Geriatric Abstracts—Asymptomatic CAD: How to Prescreen with Noninvasive Testing." *Geriatrics,* 1983, 38(9), p. 133.

97. H. A. Solomon, *The Exercise Myth* (New York: Harcourt Brace Jovanovich, 1984). Dr. Solomon devotes an entire chapter to the unreliability and risks of stress testing. He also believes the deaths and complications related to stress testing may be only "the tip of the iceberg." Because these tests are, at times, performed where preparation and supervision are not optimal, he believes many untoward events are not publicly reported.

98. J. S. Borer, et al., "Limitation of the Electrocardiographic Response to Exercise in Predicting Coronary Artery Disease," *New Engl J Med* 293 (1975): 367–71.

99. D. Scherer and M. Kaltenbach, "Frequency of Life-Threatening Complications Associated with Stress Testing," *Deutsche Medizinische Wochenschrift* 104 (1979): 1161–65. This study, from West Germany, and one of the largest ever performed, reported 1 complication in every 7,500 patients undergoing stress testing.

100. "Exercise Test Perilous for 1 in Every 9,000," *Med Tribune,* 29 July 1984. A more recent report than that in note 99, it also appeared in *Deutsche Medizinische Wochenschrift* 109 (1984): 123–27.

101. S. Snyder, "Improving the Accuracy of Interpretation of the Exercise Stress Test," *Practical Cardiology,* 1983, 9(6), pp. 55–60.

102. M. D. Meller and R. Ross, "The Risks of Exercise Stress Testing," *Practical Cardiology,* 1980, 6(1), pp. 91–100.

103. H. Nelson, "High-Tech Heart Diagnosis Studied," *Los Angeles Times* II (18 Feb. 1982): 1–2. The article quotes Dr. Daniel Berman, of the University of California, Los Angeles, Medical School, who warns that a positive result from a stress test usually leads to coronary angiography (threading a tube through the body into the heart, injecting a dye, and then taking motion picture X rays of the heart's arteries); that procedure (a common consequence of positive stress tests whether real or false) carries a risk of death in one out of every 750 patients who undergo it. He also reports that in one of every five people who undergo angiography after a supposed positive stress test result, no heart disease is found.

104. M. Udeleff, "Stress Testing Makes the Grade," *Medicenter Management* 1 (Aug./ Sept. 1984): 69–75. A cardiology technician describes how, in addition to having a "crash cart" (a table containing virtually everything that might be needed in the event of an emergency while a patient is undergoing a stress test), her facility also starts a "heparin lock" (inserting an intravenous needle in the patient to be able to inject drugs instantaneously if needed) prior to testing. She also admits to having had to inject lidocaine (a drug commonly used to help correct irregular heart rhythms or to start a heart beating that has stopped) several times while performing the stress test.

105. D. H. Spodick and R. L. Bishop, "Bundle Branch Block Induced by Exercise Testing," *Primary Cardiology,* Aug. 1984. Describes how 16 of 4,100 patients had a heart block [stopping of the heart] while undergoing a stress test.

QUESTION AND ANSWER PERIOD

Dr. Mendelsohn: I'd now like to entertain comments from those present.

Dr. Spodick: I've known Dr. Pinckney for many years and he's a great friend of mine, but I think he's got some of his figures quite wrong on the exercise test. I won't challenge him yet on the others. If you exercise normal people, the people who want to jog, you're going to get into a lot of trouble with the exercise test. That's how you can get a 40 percent accuracy figure. It depends on who you exercise and this accuracy predicted value, everything depends on the people you investigate. You take 20- to 30-year-old man—particularly an athlete, as a matter of fact, in fine condition—and you're going to get false-positive results. But you take 50- to 60-year-old people who tend to have coronary disease and you're not going to get that; you're going to get very, very few false-positive results, in fact. We exercise regularly hundreds of people between seven days and two weeks after coronary; not one of them in the last eight years has had any complications at all,* and we have been able to save them from trouble by not letting them get out of the hospital without further investigation in order to do a bypass if necessary. I'm one of the biggest critics of bypasses, so I think he's not telling you the full story, and I would only demur on that one.

Dr. Crile: I think there's an element of truth in some of the things Dr. Pinckney says, but some of the things he presents very unfairly. For example, saying a cholecystogram is 40 percent accurate in showing stones is technically true because a nonopaque stone may not visualize, but you will have a nonfunctioning gallbladder then, so you still know there's a diseased gall bladder. The test is much more accurate than he gives it credit for, although I think he is right that the sonar is coming along and becoming highly competitive with, if not replacing, the cholecystogram.

Dr. Mendelsohn: I've been using Dr. Pinckney's book for a long time now. The name of his book is *The Patient's Guide to Medical Tests* (second edition—first published in 1978 as *The Encyclopedia of Medical Tests*) by Dr. Edward and his medical editor wife Cathey Pinckney, and there are a number of other books now on the same subject that will give you the risks of medical testing and the error rate of medical tests. There's another book called *It's Your Body—Know What the Doctor Ordered: Your Complete Guide to Medical Testing,* by nurse Marion Laffey Fox and Dr. Truman G. Schnabel. As far as I'm concerned the great benefit of these books and this kind of videotape is that they're bringing before the public some of the controversies that you can see from the response here exist within medicine as to the accuracy of the tests. I think what's important is that everybody be aware of the controversy so

---

*Dr. Pinckney refers the reader to note 105.

that at least they'll be able to talk to their doctors on an intelligent level.

I mentioned earlier in the program this morning that the American Academy of Pediatrics is against the routine admission X rays on children, but as far as I know—and, Hilmon, you might know more about this than I do—as far as I know, in most hospitals they still continue to X ray adults on admission.

Professor Sorey: Right, unless there is an X ray of a certain kind. Yes, if you haven't had an X ray in the last 5 minutes, you're probably going to get X rayed again.

Dr. Mendelsohn: The X ray is taken for many reasons. The routine tuberculin skin test is now recommended to be used only in areas of a high incidence of tuberculosis. Some of us are interested in getting rid of the routine tests, the routine blood tests, urine tests, and all the rest because there are a number of studies that show now that when these tests are falsely reported back to the doctor as being positive, the doctor doesn't follow up on those tests anyway because he's so used to not looking at the results of routine tests. There's one study that I quote in my first book where they took 200 tests for syphilis and returned them as positive and only three doctors ever called up the laboratory, so I think one of the answers is to get rid of routine tests. I have to tell everybody here how surprised I was to find out that testing accounted for 50 percent of medical costs in this country. I had no idea it was that much.

The result that comes out of this kind of meeting is confusion because confusion, I think, is the beginning of knowledge, and if we have generated this kind of confusion in you then I know that we have achieved our purpose.

Lecturer's Comments

The preceding comments were sent to Dr. Pinckney for his response, which follows:

Dr. Pinckney: As to the accuracy figures of the medical tests commented upon, those figures are not mine but are taken from the medical literature; please see the *Notes* which follow my lecture. Since preparing my presentation, additional evidence has been published that makes the accuracy rate of the "stress test" even worse. Robert J. McCunney, M.D., of Boston University School of Public Health, writing in the October 1984 issue of *Occupational Health & Safety*, cites several studies that show the predictive value of that stress test to range from 5 to 46 percent, with an average accuracy rate of from only 16 to 21 percent. True, if you select people with *known* heart disease, the chance of the stress test detecting them cannot help but increase; unfortunately, medical tests are performed on patients with already known conditions or diseases, and when they are, the question of *why?* must be raised before reimbursing the cost of that test, let alone exposing the patient to the test's dangers.

As to the comment about doctors not following up on the results of the medical tests they order, there are endless reports in medical journals that reveal this persistent practice. The most recent, almost paralleling Dr. Mendelsohn's quote back in 1979, was published in 1984 in the *Southern Medical Journal* (77:1118); here, the Cleveland Clinic Foundation described how out of 2,912 patients admitted to the hospital, 75 had a positive test result for syphilis. Forty-three of those patients were never correctly evaluated; the abnormal test results were ignored.

INTRODUCTION OF THE THIRD MODERATOR

Dr. Mendelsohn: We approach our final session of Dissent in Medicine. Our third moderator, Lori Andrews, graduated Law School and took her undergraduate work at Yale. She is now a research attorney for the American Bar Foundation where she directs projects covering law and medicine. She is a member, together with John McKnight, of the Board of Directors of the People's Medical Society. In the 1940s, Milton Friedman published *Capitalism and Freedom*, in which he recommended the delicensure of doctors. Lori Andrews last year published her work *Deregulating Doctoring*, which extends, elaborates, and, in my opinion, completes the work originally done by Professor Friedman years ago. I think that decontrolling doctors is one of the most important pieces of advice for everybody involved in health issues, and I am very happy that Lori is able to be with us today. I also want to point out that Lori Andrews is author of *New Conceptions*, a book that deals with the technology surrounding the act of reproduction. She's been a guest of all the major television shows. I'm sure that those of you who haven't seen her up until now will be seeing her very frequently.

EFFECTIVENESS OF TREATMENT

Mandating Appropriate Scientific, Behavioral, and Ethical Standards— A Cardiologist Dissents

David Spodick, M.D.

INTRODUCTION OF THE SPEAKER

Lori Andrews: I've been very interested in dissent within medicine and the past day and a half's activities—hearing another viewpoint on common medical procedures and medical philosophies and hearing how the press is getting more interested in dissent in medicine and trying to round out their stories by asking people for the other side of medical issues.

I'm afraid I must say that the law is very much behind the times and hasn't even recognized that there is dissent in medicine. The law's viewpoint of medicine as a monolith is evidenced in court cases that look at the standard of care in medicine and take the majority rule in medicine as the appropriate standard of care even if the majority in medicine happens to be wrong or outdated on a particular issue.

This has been most clear to me as a result of a number of cases recently where women have refused to have cesarean sections and their doctors have gone into court, possibly at three in the morning, while the woman is in labor, and have said, "We really need a court order to force this woman to have a cesarean section against her will." The courts and judges have routinely granted these orders. The judges never consider dissent or consider the fact that there is a growing view within medicine that perhaps cesarean sections are not appropriate in all the cases for which they are recommended. And this dissenting view has been vindicated in a few instances where doctors have gotten court orders but the women escaped from them and subsequently gave birth naturally with no harm. So, I'm hoping that this conference helps focus the law's attention on the fact that there are varying viewpoints in medicine. Maybe you'll even see some beneficial changes in the legal profession.

I'm pleased to have the opportunity to introduce the speakers today. I'd like first to introduce Dr. David Spodick, who has many credentials but, more importantly, is known as "the Conscience of Cardiology." He is a professor of medicine at the University of Massachusetts Medical School and director of cardiology and noninvasive cardiology at St. Vincent Hospital. In addition to teaching at the University of Massachusetts, he is also a lecturer at the Medical School at Tufts in Boston University. He received his medical degree from the New York Medical College in 1950, and when he completed residency, he was a medical officer in the U.S. Air Force and later a special post-doctoral fellow at the National Heart Institute. He is a Fellow of the American College of Cardiology, the American College of Physicians, and the American College of Chest Physicians. He has also written for, and served on, the editorial boards of prestigious medical journals, such as *The American Journal of Cardiology, The American Heart Journal, The Archives of Internal Medicine*, and *Clinical Cardiology*. You might have noticed at the table of publications as you came in that he has several thought-provoking articles out there, including one in *The Humanist*. There he takes to task the approach of treating medicine as a miracle of the day without following up on treatments that were heralded as very important but later turned out to be harmful and faded out of medical texts with nobody closely assessing why these things happen. So, Dr. Spodick, we welcome you.

*LECTURE**

Dr. Spodick: Dr. Mendelsohn mentioned the sexist nature of medical practice. I can think of a reverse story: Two women meet and one of them says, "How's your husband?" and the other replies, "Compared to what?" That's actually what I'm going to talk about—comparisons,

---

*At the *Dissent in Medicine* meeting, a slide presentation accompanied this lecture.

comparisons of treatment. In order to know whether something you're doing for, or perhaps doing to, the patient (your victim) is worthwhile, you need a fair standard of comparison. You have to compare it with alternate treatments or with no treatment, and, to do that, you must look for the effectiveness, but also the safety, of your treatment. All medicines, in a way, are poisons—you try to poison the disease before you poison the patient. That goes for an aspirin or anything else that we take. Therefore, we want to know safety and effectiveness; and there are three aspects to this, which are always with us—the scientific, the ethical, and—I'm sorry for physicians—the behavioral. The *scientific* aim is to get a true result, and to get a true result as best we can, we need to reduce bias—and *bias* is the worst four-letter word I know. The *ethical*, which is tied up with the scientific—and all three are tied up together—is that a physician or any healer has an absolute compulsion to do his best for his patient. The question is: Does he know best? And that brings in another factor, *the quality of knowledge*. What is the quality of knowledge? How well do we know? How do we know? After all, witch doctors are ethical; they are ethical by definition, since they are doing their best. It is what they believe to be their best.

Finally, is the *behavioral* aspect, and this is the unfortunate one. Because physicians and healers have behaved poorly—either consciously or unconsciously—in the past, we need standards that compel appropriate behavior. "Appropriate behavior" means scientific *and* ethical behavior; you can't separate them. For pills and injections, the Food and Drug Administration (FDA) compels this, and it compels it only because we have many "bad actors." Therefore, the rules are very stringent. You can't bring a pill or an injection to the patient without adequate protection from the FDA. It's something I wholly approve of (even though it's made some of us squirm, and even though in some of our protocols we must give the patient four pages of a fine-print "informed consent"). But there is a form of double-standard for behavior here—both on the part of physicians and of committees in hospitals supposed to protect the patients. The double standard is: controlled clinical trials for pills and injections, yes; for surgery, no. The same hospital whose human trials committees compel FDA rules for testing a new pill will not do it for testing new surgery. Surgery has been a sacred cow. That is one of the holes in our system. However, not all is lost. Surgery can be held to the same rules. Indeed, in some cases, we have succeeded in getting it to be held to the same rules.

Now, I'm going to present some slides. The first one—a quotation—

should be clear. "If a man" (this means anybody) "will begin with certainties, he shall end in doubts. But, if he will be content to begin with doubts, he will end in certainties." This is by one of my favorite philosophers, Francis Bacon. It's not quite correct. The important thing is indeed to begin with doubts—that's what the scientist does, and he remains in doubt. But we no longer end in certainties, we only end in statistical probabilities. Moreover, today's certainty is not necessarily tomorrow's. For example, here, from a Boston newspaper in 1963 the headlines: "Asthma Licked," and "Hub Doctors Lick Asthma." Of course that bothers me, because for most of my life, I've been a Hub (that means Boston) doctor. The report reads, "A 100 percent effective treatment for asthma has been developed by two Boston physicians." One was a surgeon. To continue: "As a result, asthma can now be crossed off the list as a potential killer." Now you know! No more asthma, we're done with asthma. A Boston paper said it, Boston doctors said it. One was a famous professor of surgery, and what did he do? He snatched the glomus—a tiny organ—out of the neck. If doing it on one side didn't do it, he did the other side; if that didn't do it, his confederate gave corticosteroid treatment. Well, many of us picked up the human debris of this operation and it is no longer done (at least on adults). Like many, many other "cures" offered by top-notch people, they were ended, not by a rational clinical trial, but by trial and error—which, through the centuries, has been the way physicians tried drugs, injections, and surgery. We hope they no longer do. This operation—glomectomy— ended, mostly by trial and error.

Now, Dr. Mendelsohn referred to surveys reporting failure to tell when to do a tonsillectomy and an adenoidectomy. This slide was from the *International Hospital Tribune,* and I made this slide over 10 years ago. At that time they could not tell when to remove tonsils; they still can't tell. Here's the 1980 report of the Massachusetts Department of Health. These are areas in Massachusetts in black which show tonsillec- tomy rates over 20 percent above the statewide average, going up to 238 percent in Fairhaven. Now who's right about these? The population has about the same type of people everywhere. They still haven't decided. Tonsillectomy remains a milestone in the life of most American children.

This slide is a photo from the *Annals of Thoracic Surgery.* It follows an article on—as you see up in the right-hand corner—direct myocardial revascularization. As in many such surgical journals, there is a discussion included. (The discussion usually reflects a mutual admiration society.)

I have blacked out the name of the famous cardiac surgeon—he is thus anonymous—to protect the guilty. Now this is what he says: "So you older members may remember when I too used to present Texas-sized series to support my own new ideas, many of which did not work out fully either to my expectations or to yours." Now at the bottom, the last sentence: "I think we would be *well advised* in properly indicated cases to stick to those procedures that we *know* will work." Now think about that a little bit. Here is a distinguished surgeon, professor of surgery, who used to present "Texas-sized series" of patients (Alaska is our biggest state, but I assume Texas means something gross and big) to support his own new ideas. This means he had a lot of patients. Do large numbers mean much? Text: "Many of which did not work out fully, either to my expectation or to yours." The question to this man is: How did he get to Texas-sized before he realized he was doing more damage than good? Finally, he says, "In properly indicated cases." How did he know what was properly indicated? Obviously, he had no sure index. And then he would "stick to procedures that we *know* will work." And what was the quality of his knowledge? What is the quality of anyone's knowledge? It depends on the rules of the game, of how you get your knowledge. Fortunately, this man is no longer carving people.

Some of our false knowledge comes from what we consider to be "obvious." For example, radical breast resection for cancer of the breast—that was "obvious" since Halsted started it in the 1890s: The more you chop off, the better the patient. You know now that isn't true. Dr. Crile showed that (see Chapter 2), but I would submit to you that anybody of less than his stature couldn't have gotten away with it. Another example: High doses of insulin for diabetic ketoacidosis (diabetic coma). We now know you can do it with low doses in some cases, but it was "obvious" you had to load the medicine in. Again: Antacids for the treatment of peptic ulcers, as we'll show, "ain't necessarily so," in fact they make ulcers worse sometimes. Another: High doses of oxygen given to premature infants—it apparently caused a lot of blindness. Sympathectomy for high blood pressue—no longer done—was a big Boston operation. It also was "obvious" that an increased blood flow in the cardiac muscle (the myocardium) will improve the heart. Well, it will, but it isn't *necessarily* so. Or, that decreased cholesterol will cause improvement. Well, it may, but it isn't necessarily so. What I'm getting at is: *to the scientist, nothing is obvious.*

Here is an example. I'll try to interpret it for you. These are patients in a Boston hospital with ulcers and this is a graph of the acid in the stomach, which you're trying to reduce. As you go toward the bottom there's less acid, a fall in acid level. Levels are shown at 9 A.M., after breakfast, and in the afternoon, after lunch. These are patients on a standard, ordinary hospital diet which they could pick for themselves, and acid was reduced. In contrast are patients on a standard ulcer diet of cream, milk, etc., and you can see that the acid really doesn't budge.

Now, here's something else that Dr. Crile alluded to—the National Breast Adjuvant study. Look at those curves at the top, approximately three; there are actually five, because two are superimposed. Each of those curves is statistically equal. They are curves of survival. At the bottom are the months after mastectomy. Each curve—A, B, C, D, and E—is for different combinations of radical mastectomy, less-than-radical mastectomy, lymph node dissection, and radiation, in five different combinations. The effect on life is no different for simple or radical mastectomy in these patients. But, it had been "obvious" that taking out more breast would be "better."

Well, where are some of the "obvious" cures now? Keep in mind that in every case, the doctors performing the uncontrolled trials were enthusiastic. For coronary disease there was pericardiopexy. This was a method of putting powder into the pericardial sac around the heart and letting adhesions form, which they proposed would cause new blood vessels to grow into the heart. But, when they cut the adhesions, they bled from the cardiac end—the blood was going the wrong way. Another, the Vineberg implant: hundreds of thousands, maybe millions of these were done for coronary disease in Canada, the United States, and a lot of other countries. It is not being done anymore; it's a no-good operation. Omentopexy is another.

Another was internal mammary ligation—that was the "quick and dirty" way to solve coronary disease. All that was needed, under local anesthesia, was two little incisions on each side of the sternum to permit tying off the internal mammary arteries, which would, in theory, divert blood into the heart. You should have seen the results: They were marvelous in many cases. Hundreds of thousands of such operations were done all over the world. Yet, two controlled trials shot this "quick fix" down.

There was also gastropexy for "dropped stomach" and nephropexy for "dropped kidney." Once there were special X rays in the 1930s, used to tell some people that if they had pain in the stomach, the stomach had "dropped." If they had pain in the back, their kidneys had "dropped," or their ovaries. (In the 1920s, they said that dancing the Charleston had shaken the ovaries out of their beds and they may have "dropped.") Lots of money was made on this, but you don't hear about it anymore. You don't hear about those terrible operations for so-called "tipped-womb," for ladies who had pain in the back and other symptoms. The womb can be happy in almost any position.

Here is a slide that I made from government figures: the death rate curve of coronary disease. It starts in 1950 and rises in all categories of the population until roughly 1967. Then there is a sharp break and death rates come sharply down. Coronary disease mortality—the death rate— has been falling, falling, falling, and it's still falling. It's about 40 percent now, below the peak. Now consider this: If, in the middle 1960s you had developed your own pet treatment, an immunization, let's say, for coronary disease, you could have administered it to the vast majority of the population, and if you'd gone around and done that just before the death rates sharply turned around, you would have earned the Nobel Prize. You'd have been "responsible" for the "breakthrough"—all that *unless you had done a controlled study,* a study in which half your patients couldn't get your treatment. Then half of your patients would have had exactly the death rate that the "immunized" half had. That is one of the main reasons for doing controlled trials. Time changes disease. That's called *time bias*.

I'm sorry Dr. Crile isn't here, but I think he is quite aware that the appendectomy for appendicitis that he mentioned yesterday refers to a different disease now than it did in the days when appendicitis meant pus in the appendix. There's much less apendicitis and they usually do not have pus in the appendix nowadays. Now appendicitis probably is a viral disease.

We asked before: Does reducing cholesterol actually help? Well, it may in some people. But look at a drug which is still on the market in a World Health Organization cooperative trial. They gave this drug over a period of 9.6 years (in fact, there's a new report a month ago after a total of 13.6 years). What this shows is the drug, clofibrate, given against placebo. The clofibrate was given to a high-cholesterol group, patients in danger; the placebo was given to a high-cholesterol and to a low-cholesterol group. Notice that death from all causes was higher in the clofibrate group than in the placebo group. *But it reduced cholesterol.* Now, reduction of cholesterol may very well be beneficial, but this agent may not be the one to use for most people. That's what the results say. So, getting a reduced cholesterol will satisfy the laboratory. The controlled trial doesn't ask that question. It asks, "What happens to the patient?"

Does increasing coronary blood flow necessarily increase oxygen to the heart? It can, and they do it in the coronary operations, but not with this drug, dipyridamole, which was advertised to do that. If the same kind of experiment is done with ordinary, common, cheap, everyday nitroglycerin, used by millions and millions of angina sufferers, coronary blood flow didn't increase but the heart received more oxygen. You don't have to increase blood flow, though it's nice to do it. The point is that a controlled trial of both of these agents shows that nitroglycerin works and dipyridamole doesn't. The controlled trial does not ask what the laboratory is going to find. It asks, "What happened to the patient?" Thirty years ago, common nitroglycerin "had" to be a coronary vaso-dilator to explain its effects. Now, every cardiologist knows that it *can* be but *wasn't* in this case—that it doesn't need that mechanism.

Now here's a study, from the *American Journal of Cardiology*, of that "quick and dirty" operation in which in a few minutes you could tie off the internal mammary arteries under local anesthesia with no operative mortality, and the patients—lo and behold—got better. This was a study of 304 supposedly unselected patients—a large group. These patients were largely "better" and the electrocardiogram improved in 64 percent—very objective. Indeed, it became normal in 13 percent. But uncontrolled, very enthusiastic, in an authoritative journal, and 304 patients. Now, the nice thing about the controlled trial is that it allows for the natural tendency of most diseases to get better.

But here is a *controlled* trial, from the *New England Journal of Medicine*, of only 17 patients with angina, in which they had only skin incisions and no arteries tied. (This was done in 1959. You couldn't do just a skin incision today, because you need full disclosure.) The people who had only skin incisions and did not have tying off of the vessels did just as well or better as those who did. In fact, their average exercise tolerance, in minutes on a treadmill, improved more than those who had the "real" operation. Well, internationally, there were 152 published uncontrolled reports of it, all 152 enthusiastic. Thousands of people had this, maybe tens of thousands; but there were only two well controlled trials. I showed you one. Is that operation being done? It is not being done now. Its ineffectiveness was demonstrated in quite small numbers of patients. Do big numbers mean anything? Well, although 100 zeros are very impressive on paper, they are no more than a single zero.

Skepticism is the highest of duties of the scientist, and blind faith the one unpardonable sin. This goes mostly for the true scientist who is a true humanitarian and is skeptical, above all, of his *own* work and is ready to discard tomorrow what he said today. He wants proof.

It is possible that you don't always have to do control studies. If I see you with a bleeding artery, I know very well that it is highly likely that if I don't tie that artery off, you're going to die—I don't need a contolled study. There are some conditions in which the patient or the natural history of disease is an appropriate control—as in rare diseases, diseases with a high early mortality, diseases in one of paired organs. Historically, for example, iron for iron-deficiency anemia, very clearly, is an open and shut case. But very few things in medicine are that way: vitamin B_{12} for pernicious anemia, streptomycin for tuberculous meningitis, penicillin for most bacterial endocarditis (which was almost totally fatal before penicillin), and insulin for diabetes mellitus. But, as Dr. Crile indicated yesterday, historical controls are very misleading when you use what you remember of patients' histories or look through your files. They nearly always beget "success," and even when they come out the same way as in a controlled trial, the success rate is usually much greater. They're biased.

Biases can be unconscious or conscious. Bias in which the physician or the investigator slants his or her results is *conscious bias*. Such investigators bias their work. We have had many such buccaneers, but there are many fewer of them since the creation of the FDA. Then there is *time bias*. Look at the changing disease scene: coronary disease with its mortality; appendicitis is a different disease today, rarely pus in the appendix; changing disease severity, as in acute rheumatic fever. That was a much worse disease than it is now; indeed we hardly see it. A few years ago, I was a visiting professor in South Africa where you see differences in the population. Obviously, for the whites it is like ours, but the blacks have a miserable time with acute rheumatic fever.

Now, what about experts? This slide is from *Harper's Bazaar*, not the Sears, Roebuck catalog: an electric corset. The small print says how marvelous it is for rheumatism, paralysis, numbness, dyspepsia, liver, kidney, and so forth; recommended by Dr. W. A. Hammond of New York, the late "Surgeon General of the United States." There's an expert for you. He endorsed this thing and they'll even send it to you, postpaid, on trial. Marvelous. And the name—"Pall Mall Electric Association"—

in London. Imported! Well, this is to indicate that intellect and skill are irrelevant here, excepting when an evaluation is carried out appropriately. Intellect, skill, status, and expertise are no guarantee that you're getting something good, as with the "Hub Doctors" mentioned earlier.

Here was a controlled trial that threw out something by one of the finest surgeons in the country—gastric freezing for ulcers. A freezing solution was put through the stomach. There was a distinguished innovator, Owen Wangensteen, one of the finest surgeons ever. He reported this in a distinguished forum—the Moynihan Lecture, the yearly prize lecture, at the Royal College of Surgeons in London (not many Americans are invited to do that). He "succeeded": 841 patients in ten hospitals; no controls. Marvelous. They then sold 2,500 freezing machines in this country alone. Yet, you don't hear about that anymore because it's not being done. Shortly thereafter, a young, fairly unknown man studied 160 patients in five hospitals in a randomized trial. They were randomized so that about half would receive gastric freezing and half had a sham procedure using tap water. There was no significant difference in the ulcers between one and one half years and 24 months. He shot down gastric freezing, and, to his credit, Dr. Wangensteen admitted he was wrong. So, the status of the investigator doesn't guarantee anything. It's how you do it.

The randomized controlled trial is nearly universally applicable. It can be designed for *almost* anything. Not everything. It seeks a true result, irrespective of hypothesis. (Hypothesis: that low cholesterol is necessarily good; hypothesis: that increasing blood flow in the heart is necessarily effective.) It does not examine hypotheses. These change and may be wrong. The randomized trial bypasses the prejudices of both the doctor *and the patient*. It minimizes many biases, and it ensures—it compels—scientific, and therefore ethical, behavior.

Many physicians, especially surgeons, recognize the randomized controlled trial in principle but violate it in practice, and they are at the top of the profession. Indeed, they are people I personally respect and often personally know, but the approach is wrong and they have to admit that. Because they say it but they don't do it, it is Orwellian. Surgery still remains a sacred cow—even though the coronary bypass operation has been subjected to controlled trials and is finding its place.

So, this double-thinking brings us to the behavioral aspect of treatment. Let's just give examples of poor behavior by physicians: Prescriptions despite lack of efficacy; diethylstilbesterol (DES) for habitual abortion; diet in acute peptic ulcer, which is almost irrelevant; bedrest in acute viral hepatitis; prejudice, prejudging efficacy; diversion of patients from studies, principally by physicians; bias in patient assignment; counseling nonparticipation in trials; no concern with methodology. (The latter behavior is indicated by the World Conference of Gastronenterology, where 3,000 people went to the session featuring people claiming to have the best operation while only 300 went to the session on how to determine the best operation.)

Here's another example of poor behavior: In three decades, mortality (the death rate) of people with bleeding ulcers was unchanged. Yet the amount of surgery for bleeding ulcers increased—with no effect, yet they continued to do more operations.

Here's something more recent, from 1979. This is a report, the first report, of a bypass operation during acute myocardial infarction ("a coronary"). What they did was to compare patients who had the coronary bypass with patients who had medical treatment, and they had marvelous results. They looked at the results only after the treatments were completed—what we call a retrospective study. *There were no concurrent control patients.* These people reported again in the *Journal of the American College of Cardiology* in 1984. They said the same thing they said before, so I wrote a letter to the editor. I said that in 1979, they declared that, although the data were promising, a controlled randomized trial would be necessary to resolve this issue. But they didn't do it. They answered that more than two years ago their group voted to begin randomized trials, but that they had difficulty with funding because of the position taken by administrators of their medical centers that the trial should be totally funded and paid for. I can't evaluate their motivations. They still didn't do an appropriate clinical trial, yet they still claim it ought to be done. This is a form of double-think. (I hate to say hypocrisy, because they may well be telling the truth.) But they waited to even suggest voting to do what they promised to do in the beginning. The solution is that on the first day of a new treatment, they should have mandated for their surgical treatment exactly what is mandated for a pill or an injection—a controlled trial starting with patient number one.

Here is something published in the August 1984 *Journal of the American College of Cardiology*, a report of the principal investigators of the CASS (Coronary Artery Surgery Study) and their associates, of randomized and randomizable patients. I want to call your attention to the fact that 1,319 patients—in other words, almost twice as many as got into the study—were not randomized. They were offered it but declined as a result of *physician refusal* in 69 percent. Their physicians would not consent. When the study ended, they showed that for this kind of patient it didn't make any difference whether you treated them medically or surgically at that time. But the point is that almost twice as many as entered the study were counseled by the physicians not to get into it— into a study—*to find out how good (or bad) it was*. That is what I object to. Not that it is a bad operation per se.

Once again, just to emphasize the lesson, I consider a randomized controlled trial to be the optimum method of evaluating therapy. *Scientifically,* it minimizes biases, objective and subjective. *Behaviorally,* it ensures, *it compels,* honest practice. *Ethically,* it mandates truthful recruitment—you have to tell the patient what you're doing. If it is new, you have to tell them, "Well, we just started; we have to get the bugs out." How many do you think will volunteer under those conditions if they had truthful, informed consent for surgery? After all, technically, it takes time to improve most surgery.

Now, I will finish with something different. Because DES was referred to, I'm going to tell you what the *real* DES scandal was. DES (diethylstilbesterol) was advanced to prevent habitual abortion and other accidents of pregnancy on the basis of seven early studies in which there were no real controls. There were a couple of contrived controls and a couple of historical controls. That is what established DES and what led to more than 50,000 women a year getting DES until the FDA put a stop to it in the seventies. Now, can you blame the physicians for not knowing that *one generation later* there would be trouble? I can't blame them for that. Nobody could predict that. Now, I'll show you what you *can* blame them for—the *real* DES scandal. During the same period there were six studies in which there were controls of a quality from reasonably good to excellent; three of the studies were blinded. Their results were all negative. Now, the physicians learning about DES had in the same literature these references: a group of poor studies saying "yes" and a group of high-quality studies saying "no." Those who administered DES accepted the enthusiastic reports. That's the real DES scandal.

Finally, regarding the case of surgery, which is my main point today: Surgery has been a sacred cow, and probably we'll always have sacred cows. The important thing is to control the sacred cowboys who milk them and market the products.

I began by citing my favorite English philosopher. Here is my favorite

American philosopher, Will Rogers: "It's not what we don't know that causes trouble. It's what we know that ain't so." That is the basis for the randomized control trial. Thank you.

QUESTION AND ANSWER PERIOD

Q: I have to ask you, Dr. Spodick, for your speculations on why physicians who presumably have been trained in the scientific method for so many years pay so little attention to it once they get out of school. Is it possibly because they pay so little attention to it in school?

Dr. Spodick: That may possibly be it, part of the tradition of medicine, and the physician who has set himself up—and also patients set physicians up—as a god. There's the Hippocratic background, which makes you that way. I think little attention was given to this sort of thing. Keep in mind that the physician is just like the rest of you, only with special training, and we physicians all have human failings. I think it was almost lucky that in the middle part of this century money came into medicine, as it never did before, to involve research. The nonmedical scientist got in the game and wanted to get a fair result, a true result, to eliminate bias. The physician's ethical compulsion to do what he thought was best for his patient, like the witchdoctor, led to what his own inbred ways led him to do—and he'd been trained that he was an end in himself—a physician's decision to do something on whatever basis was "okay" was legal.

I think the students we have today are so much better than the old-timers. There's a lot less arrogance. There's a lot more humility, because the scientist is essentially a humble man; he looks down and sees his own clay feet. But he may have clay feet with a good structure on top, and that's what we want to find out. I think since there's been less arrogance, we're getting a more and more scientific approach. The only thing is, and I still don't understand it, that we tolerate the double-standard behavior with regard to surgery.

The fact is that you can apply the same rules to both medical and surgical treatments, but it's been done so late with certain surgical procedures that it is difficult to get physicians to tell their patients to get into surgical trials. They've already become convinced. So, as usual, we are backing into the future. The point is, on the first day of a new treatment, or the new application of an old treatment, you don't know whether it is good or bad.

Q: Dr. Spodick, there has been a proposal that was published in a Yale law journal last year that surgery be regulated in the same way that drugs are, that there be an agency that deals with the introduction of surgery, and that only a few centers be allowed to try out a new operation and that it be done in a controlled study. I read that and I thought that the idea that it could actually get accepted by the medical profession was a bit far-fetched. Do you think something like that is worth pushing for so that there isn't the wide-scale adoption of particular procedures based on the status of an individual proposing it? Would you be in favor of something along those lines? Do you think it sort of an ethical responsiblity of the profession rather than the law to encourage something like that?

Dr. Spodick: That's a very difficult question. I've always disliked external compulsion—except in the case of the FDA; bureaucratic as it is, it's been a net benefit. I think that all treatments should be ultimately subjected to the same kinds of tests and, since that can be done and has been done, I'd like to see the details of that but I certainly feel it's in the right direction.

Q: I think randomized controls are very important. I'd like to suggest, though, that in many instances I think that time has come. There are new developments, and I refer particularly to the computer, which can do studies, if properly fed, considerably better than randomized trials can, because randomized trials in themselves, as you mention, can also be biased. For example—and I believe, by the way, that I think one of the salvations for the medical profession will be the engineers—I've worked with two graduates of MIT who are also M.D.s. One suggested, for example, that in treating breast cancer it's possible to take 21 different modalities and, by a retrospective study, comparing in literally hundreds and hundreds of cases how each combination of these 21 modalities with each different treatment, surgical or nonsurgical, could be thrown up in a recognizable pattern. Thus, you can actually get a comparison of results instantly by simply reviewing the charts, or by doing a prospective study as well. Now, the advantage is that then a doctor could simply list for each patient the 21 different modalities and varieties of location and so forth in breast cancer and get all possible combinations and all possible treatments for each possible combination—something which the human mind could never do alone. This is such a good idea that he couldn't get funding for it, but I'd like to suggest that in the future that will be perhaps a better method than the attempts at randomized studies which are also limited now by legal, moral, and ethical considerations.

Dr. Spodick: I cannot agree that it's an engineering solution. That is a deus ex machina of a kind which, I think you know, is subject to the common equation "garbage in, garbage out." You have to know the quality of what goes in. Historical data are very, very difficult. You did mention "prospectively," but you still have the follow-up of the patient, in order to really know what happens, and our labs are imperfect, our hypotheses are imperfect, and the real result is *what happens to the patient in the long run.* I'm sorry he didn't get money for it. Maybe he could not design a study which would give it a fair trial. Because, if it is better, that's what we want. I don't reject anything out of hand. I don't reject acupuncture. I want a fair study. I do not believe that you can, as we say, dredge the data—that is, take a computer which remembers far better than any of us and can put a lot of things together and predict the result—without actually doing it, and thereby see what would happen. And ethically, morally, and legally, you must give your patient half a chance not to receive the treatment.

Q: Contrary to "garbage in" and "garbage out" is "quality in" and "quality out," and I would point out that if you look at a medical journal, which is all we have to go by today, the human mind can see a treatment in two ways—e.g., the size of the lesion against the length of survival, or the pregnancy or nonpregnancy against the length of survival—and can only take a few of these at a time. The machine can indeed interpret and, just as if the human mind were capable of taking in all the evidence that you wish to consider, the machine can do that and, if properly fed, will provide very valuable information.

Dr. Spodick: What if your new treatment is worse than the disease? I'm talking about a new treatment now. You can't know that unless you try it out, and you can't ethically or morally offer it unless you give your patient half a chance not to receive it. In addition to which, much of the material generated by physicians is of dubious quality, as you can see. There are biases in many, many cases. I would rather have a field test with a randomized trial.

Q: You can give field tests, but with all the field tests and the randomized trials that you said, you couldn't tell what was going to happen a generation later in any case. And you do have to actually treat either a few animals or a few people, but from the result of that you can then get a much greater evaluation of your figures. Actually, you can take thousands of cases treated by many, many different people in many areas. You can localize certain information, and some can be cast out and not put in the computer. But all I'm suggesting is that the computer is going to be an additional tool of medicine that will be much more valuable.

Dr. Spodick: An additional tool, meaning prognostically if you don't intervene. It still doesn't test the intervention. Prognostically maybe. But you also have another problem. Material from many different people isn't necessarily the same material unless they are under a rigid protocol like the CASS study, where everybody is under a quality assurance center and all of it goes in the same way. We've had too much experience with medical evidence and we're getting around that right now. Your proposal for the computer is fine as far as it goes—for organizing material, showing relationships that we can't tell on our own, perhaps giving a prognosis. But when it comes to treatment, the intervention *has to be tried.* The patients also have to be given a chance not to get it or to get alternate treatment.

Q: I question it from your own slides. I know the doctor you mentioned, the cardiologist who became a lawyer. As a young thoracic surgeon, I sat through the thoracic surgical meetings and I heard him and a dozen others every year present hundreds and hundreds and thousands of cases treated a certain way and randomized.

Dr. Spodick: He randomized patients? I have to have the proof of that. To my knowledge he never did.

Q: Just a minute, I'm not saying he did it necessarily, but I say in the various papers presented. The next year, the operation which was so wonderful and proven, you never heard about it. There was a new operation that the same people, and this man in particular, would come up with for cardiac surgery, and the thousands of people who had died on the previous operation were forgotten; there were another thousand here. I think the individual trying to judge his own work, even with randomized samples, is biased. Again, I knew Owen Wangensteen, a marvelous man, and I was out there as his guest professor as a young man when he was freezing stomachs, and I thought to myself, "He's going to freeze a stomach and it's going to break"—and that's what really ended his work, not the randomized trials. Several of the otherwise normal patients' frozen stomachs literally cracked and fell apart, and they died. That was what happened and that's what made him change his mind. So, as you say, the individual brilliant man can just be biased, although not wanting to be. But if you can throw in enough cases and enough individuals doing the work and if it can be analyzed in an objective way—and it can be by computer—I think you'll get much better results.

Dr. Spodick: "Objective way?" All our statistical tests are fitted to an objective model which includes true randomization, not the kind by that surgeon you and I mentioned. My recollection is different from yours. There were no true randomizations. The true ones came in with the coronary bypass—when they were forced to do it rather late in the game. When the man says that something is "at random," that's not the same. I don't want to belabor this audience with that, but my recollection is quite different from yours on that, and I think I have the data.

Q: Perfusion of the blood to the heart and muscles for angina pectoris was introduced by the homeopathic school in 1857, and it still survives as one of the only tried and true pharmacological treatments of any heart condition. I don't usually talk about this, but homeopathic medicine* was my first love and remains a big love of mine and I've often thought that it would be a good idea if physicians today were to investigate the way in which the homeopathic school did ascertain the pharmacological mechanisms of action and efficacy of certain drugs. The use of nitroglycerin is not the only one that they introduced which is still in use today. There are quite a number of others still in use in orthodox medicine.

Dr. Spodick: There are many that are not. I have a background in homeopathy, too, and I reject most of it. Like kali bichromicum for a discharging ear, or atropine for scarlet fever; I'd rather use penicillin. I'd be very careful about that. On the other hand, homeopaths do very little harm because the dilutions they use are so great. I think there's a lot to be said for that because there's a natural tendency in a patient toward improvement and therefore it's important that you don't lose that natural tendency by poisoning with medicines. The reason that Samuel Hahnemann's patients survived was that he used very little medicine, while his competitors in southern Germany, who ran him out of the country, were poisoning patients. In the last century and the early part of this century, homeopathy was a great saver of lives. (Do you know what the most commonly used medicine was in the first century in this country? It was

---

*Homeopathy is a system of therapeutics founded by Samuel Hahnemann [1755–1843] in which disease are treated by drugs that are capable of producing in healthy persons symptoms like those of the disease to be treated.

calomel—mercurous chloride—taken internally and often in large doses.) Homeopathic patients survived and they have contributed mightily to medicine. But I would disagree with you on many of the items.

Q: Dr. Spodick, I never heard of a division for noninvasive cardiology. It sounds like a good place for a man with a recommendation for coronary bypass surgery to go.

Dr. Spodick: No, no, "noninvasive" diagnostic. Noninvasive cardiology is where we do not penetrate the skin, and every hospital has it. Electrocardiograms, for an old example.

Q: It's just diagnostic, you mean. . . .

Dr. Spodick: It is just diagnostic. Our biggest item today is the echocardiogram, with which we are constantly diagnosing things you couldn't tell without it. And it's no pain or strain for the patient; that's the main thing.

Q: Where would you suggest a patient go, knowing that coronary bypass surgery is overdone. Where would you suggest people go for a second opinion?

Dr. Spodick: Well, second opinion is always a problem, because if you got a third opinion, you might get two going one way and another going the other way. There is an important set of indications for coronary bypass surgery. The CASS study showed that in some patients you didn't have to go right to it. I would only say to you that the major medical centers probably will have people of varying degrees of certainty in a particular case. My view is that, in general, in the major medical centers, it's been indicated. But I cannot tell you one from another, because we all differ among ourselves in these things.

Q: In other words, if you went to a place like New York University, which does a high volume of those operations, that might be a good place to be if you truly needed the operation. But if you're going to find out if you should have it, that might not be the place to go.

Dr. Spodick: Well, that's possible. I told Dr. Cooley at a meeting once—and you know he's an outstandingly excellent surgeon who does more than anyone else in this field—that I'd be delighted for him to do my coronaries if someone else tells him I need it. What I think is that you need a conservative cardiologist. But conservative cardiologists utilize the operation, too.

I'm a conservative cardiologist. But I think the bypass is indicated in a fair number of people. People with left main coronary disease have to have it—it's almost a medical emergency. People with symptoms and whom all the medicine we know doesn't help may need it. The approach of Pritikin with diet seems to cure angina in a lot of people who otherwise are not cured by medicines; maybe that's a good one.

Q: First of all, I'd just like to echo one thing that you said, and that is that anytime you do a restrospective study, be it with computer or any other means, it implies that you have an understanding and knowledge of all the variables that could possibly be relevant to that particular case, and if you don't have a knowledge of all the possible variables, then a retrospective study cannot give any conclusive results. Secondly, I'd like to ask you to give us your ideas of the selection process for what particular methods of therapy should be selected for randomized studies. A lot of people in this audience are involved in one way or another with a variety of unorthodox therapies and, generally speaking, I think the medical profession as a whole misses a big opportunity in that people are going to participate in or go to those unorthodox therapies whether or not the medical practitioner suggests that they do so or recommends strongly that they don't. In those instances, would it not be of greater advantage to match those individuals with individuals undergoing standard orthodox medical therapy and then utilize that patient population rather than alienate it?

Dr. Spodick: There's an excellent point. I think that's very definitely so. If a reasonable kind of treatment is advocated and unorthodox, and it appears to be safe, we have to say it *appears* to be safe. In addition, often unorthodox treatments are much less expensive. There are people who say they feel better, and we have to allow for a natural tendency to improve. I would definitely agree with you on that and we should not reject anybody's approach out of hand. That even goes for chiropractic for some things. I don't know anything about it, but I certainly think that anything that people will go to—you made an excellent point that hadn't occurred to me: People will go to these things if the doctor fails them, and, to a patient, it's how he or she feels that counts. If a person feels better, the practitioner has done something for him or her. That goes for every kind of therapy. I think that's just an excellent point; that's one of the best reasons to actually look into unorthodox treatments.

Q: I have a small question about the randomization issue. If you possibly would consider using people who would go to alternate medical procedures as controls, I would question whether or not the two populations would be the same.

Dr. Spodick: No, no, no. The randomization usually overcomes that.

Q: In other words, how do you choose your control? Statistics happens to be my field. . . .

Dr. Spodick: You don't select. Statistics are only strong in relation to the design of the experiment. It's relatively simple. You take a group of people you would treat with whatever treatment you're testing. They all have the same criteria. Those are the known variables. This gentleman referred to the unknown variables, which you can't get out of history; you must go forward. You then use a statistically determined table of randomization, which forces you to assign the patients in a previously unknown order either to treatment or to being controls. What randomization does is take the choice out of the hands of the doctor and makes chance alone determine who gets which treatment. So, since you started with patients who are matched for the known variables—the things you'd send them for treatment for anyway—randomization is supposed to, and usually does, equally distribute the unknown variables.

We don't know what the patient's genetics are, we don't know what other things are going on in a person, so we match what we do know when we use randomization, and randomization forces the patients into two groups absolutely separated from the doctor's biases.

Q: Right. I appreciate that, you've described it very well. My question referred to the usefulness of considering people who would not choose the surgery as any kind of controls. You see, as I'm sure you're aware, there would be very many variables that might be different.

Dr. Spodick: Very true, and we can't overcome everything. Science, ethics, and humanity compel us to *do our best*. We have to try to assume and try to find out what is best, and we have to get our knowledge beyond the state of that famous surgeon who committed so much carnage.

Q: Dr. Spodick, we've all heard many doctors say something like, "It's all in your head, go home and take an aspirin," and the joke that you had, the cartoon on the screen that indicated a Harvard graduate dressed as a witchdoctor—maybe there's more truth to it than we would suppose. Dr. Sheldon Deall, President of the International Congress of Applied Kinesiology, who has the Swan Clinic in Tucson, Arizona, indicated there is a tremendous weight of evidence that the ritual of medicine convinces the patient that something is occurring and, whether you have a controlled study or not, some of them are going to get better in spite of the drug; and some who get better with the drug get better not because of the drug but because of some psychological manifestation. As some say, the mind heals. To what extent can you displace or separate this psychological effect from actually testing the drug?

Dr. Spodick: But that is why you have a control group. The control group may get a placebo, which isn't exactly no treatment. We assume that psychological factors occur to the same extent in the placebo group as in the group that gets the active treatment. The doctor is blinded to which one each gets.

Q: But, to what extent can you determine whether or not some are more amenable to this hypnotic ritual suggestion than others that are not?

Dr. Spodick: What you're saying is quite true, although this idea that "it's all in your head" is something that most modern doctors reject. There are kooks, but if a person says he has a headache, he has a headache, though there may be no disease in his head.

Q: I would just like to point out to the audience the difficulty of setting up some of these experiments. About 10 years ago, my son was an intern and he got involved in a discussion of breast and bottle feeding with a pediatric resident, and the pediatric resident said, "I won't believe that breast feeding is better until I see a prospective controlled triple-blind study"—one in which neither the doctor, nor the mother, nor the baby knows whether it's getting the breast or the bottle.

Dr. Spodick: It's a good joke, but there are ways around that. You can't blind a person to surgery, and we don't do sham incisions today. You just blind the people who score your study as to how is the baby doing, to what the baby received. They haven't seen it and the baby obviously doesn't have an opinion at this point, and that's the way you would get around it. It makes a good story, but it's certainly not relevant.

Dr. Mendelsohn: Well, I agree, David, it's a good story and I'm going to repeat it, giving you full credit. I know that we have to move on, but before you leave I wanted to bring up this question of why the FDA has been willing to submit, has been eager to submit, drugs but not surgery to control study. I notice that you had the Dieckman study on your list of DES studies, and I was part of that study at the University of Chicago under Dieckman, Hasseltine, and Davis. That was done in the late 1940s and it was concluded about '50 or '51. I was sure at that point, as a medical student, that once the University of Chicago Medical School determined by means of a controlled study, that DES was no good, that it was useless, that nobody in the country would ever use it. Well, of course, what happened was that 6 million women received DES between 1940 and 1980.

Today, there are two procedures that are in the newspapers. The first was recently when Dr. Gunnar Stickler for the Mayo Clinic's Department of Pediatrics, came out against tympanostomy, the operation where they put tubes in the ears, pointing out that four controlled studies now all show that tympanostomy is no good. This is an operation that's been done on more than a million children a year for the last 15 years or so. The second is the study from Bogota, Colombia, challenging the neonatal intensive care centers where they're taking premature babies, weighing between 1 and 2.5 kilograms and, instead of putting them into the high-tech, star-wars nurseries, they are binding them to their mothers, thus using the mother's heat as the natural incubator instead of the isolette and letting the infants nurse whenever they want using a very simplified formula. They're getting survival results that are at least as good as those of the most expensive neonatal intensive care units. So what I'd like is your own speculation about how surgery has remained exempt for a half a century. How come we, you and I, who are nonoperating doctors, have to knuckle under while the surgeons ride high and mighty?

Dr. Spodick: It's double-standard behavior. This is 1984 and surgeons, of course, are often the tail that wags the dog, even in the best hospitals. They bring in money. I can't assign motivations, but hospital committees do it one way for the nonsurgeons and another for the surgeons, and they make up these nonsensical stories about how it's unethical to randomize, or having to perfect the technique. But I have demonstrated, in an article in the *American Journal of Cardiology*, that you can perfect the technique and do a controlled study at the same time. It's entirely possible. But we must compel *equal standards*. Every little doc could do his own thing until the FDA came in; every drug company could do its own thing until the FDA came in. I think perhaps Ms. Andrews has the answer—that legalistically we have to compel decent behavior. You would then see how soon it becomes more than a matter of ritual—the ritual of putting the statement in your paper, "We must do it, but I'm not going to do it." Ritual without reverence is mockery.

IMMUNIZATIONS

A Dissenting View

Richard Moskowitz, M.D.

INTRODUCTION OF THE SPEAKER

Lori Andrews: Thank you. Next, we'll be hearing from Dr. Richard Moskowitz, who will talk to us about immunizations. Dr. Moskowitz graduated Phi Beta Kappa from Harvard University and received his medical degree at New York University, but he has not taken a narrow-minded approach to his professional interest. From 1963 to 1965 he was a graduate fellow in the department of philosophy at the University of Colorado graduate school. He studied homeopathy in Athens, Greece, as well as at the National Center for Homeopathy in Washington, D.C., where he currently serves as the director of publications and is a member of the permanent teaching faculty. He has also practiced in a variety of settings. He was the founder and medical director of the Boulder Free Clinic and a volunteer physician on the Medical Committee for Human Rights in New York. He's now in the private practice of classical homeopathy and has published extensively in journals such as *Homeopathy Today*, *Homeotherapy*, and *The Journal of the American Institute of Homeopathy*. Thank you, Dr. Moskowitz.

LECTURE

Dr. Moskowitz: For the past 10 years or so, I have felt a deep and growing compunction against giving routine immunizations to children. It began with the fundamental belief that people have the right to make that choice for themselves. Soon I discovered that I could no longer bring myself to give the injections even when the parents wished me to.

At bottom, I have always felt that the attempt to eradicate entire microbial species from the biosphere must inevitably upset the balance of nature in fundamental ways that we can as yet scarcely imagine. Such concerns loom ever larger as new vaccines continue to be developed, seemingly for no better reason than that we have the technical capacity to make them and thereby to demonstrate our power, as a civilization, to manipulate the evolutionary process itself.

Purely from the viewpoint of our own species, even if we could be sure that the vaccines were harmless, the fact remains that they are compulsory, that all children are required to undergo them without any sensitive regard for basic differences in individual susceptibility, to say nothing of the wishes of the parents or the children themselves.

Most people can readily accept the fact that, from time to time, certain laws that some of us strongly disagree with may be necessary for the public good. But the issue in this case involves nothing less than the introduction of foreign proteins or even live viruses into the bloodstream of entire populations. For that reason alone, the public is surely entitled to convincing proof, beyond any reasonable doubt, that artificial immunization is in fact a safe and effective procedure, in no way injurious to health, and that the threat of the corresponding natural diseases remains sufficiently clear and urgent to warrant mass inoculation of everyone, even against their will if necessary.

Unfortunately, such proof has never been given; and, even if it could be, continuing to employ vaccines against diseases that are no longer prevalent or no longer dangerous hardly qualifies as an emergency.

Finally, even if such an emergency did exist, and artificial immunization could be shown to be an appropriate response to it, the decision would remain essentially a *political* one, involving issues of public health and safety that are far too important to be settled by any purely scientific or technical criteria, or indeed by *any* criteria less authoritative than the clearly articulated sense of the community about to be subjected to it.

For all of these reasons, I want to present the case against routine immunization as clearly and forcefully as I can. What I have to say is not quite a formal theory capable of rigorous proof or disproof. It is simply an attempt to explain my own experience, a nexus of interrelated facts, observations, reflections and hypotheses which, taken together, are more or less coherent and plausible and make intuitive sense to me.

I offer them to the public in part because the growing refusal of parents to vaccinate their children is so seldom articulated or taken seriously. The fact is that we have been taught to accept vaccination as a sort of involuntary communion, a sacrament of our own participation in the unrestricted growth of scientific and industrial technology, utterly heedless of the long-term consequences to the health of our own species, let alone to the balance of nature as a whole. For that reason alone, the other side of the case urgently needs to be heard.

1. Are the Vaccines Effective?

There is widespread agreement that the time period since the common vaccines were introduced has seen a remarkable decline in the incidence and severity of the corresponding natural infections. But the customary assumption that the decline is *attributable* to the vaccines remains unproven, and continues to be seriously questioned by eminent authorities in the field. The incidence and severity of whooping cough, for example, had already begun to decline precipitously long before the pertussis vaccine was introduced,[1] a fact which led the epidemiologist C. C. Dauer to remark, as far back as 1943:

> If mortality (from pertussis) continues to decline at the same rate during the next 15 years, it will be extremely difficult to show statistically that (pertussis immunization) had any effect in reducing mortality from whooping cough.[2]

Much the same is true not only of diphtheria and tetanus, but also of TB, cholera, typhoid, and other common scourges of a bygone era, which began to disappear toward the end of the nineteenth century, perhaps partly in response to improvements in public health and sanitation, but in any case long before antibiotics, vaccines, or any specific medical measures designed to eradicate them.[3]

Reflections such as these led the great microbiologist René Dubos to observe that microbial diseases have their own natural history, independent of drugs and vaccines, in which asymptomatic infection and symbiosis are far more common than overt disease:

It is barely recognized, but nevertheless true, that animals and plants, as well as men, can live peacefully with their most notorious microbial enemies. The world is obsessed by the fact that poliomyelitis can kill and maim several thousand unfortunate victims every year. But more extraordinary is the fact that millions upon millions of young people become infected by polio viruses, yet suffer no harm from the infection. The dramatic episodes of conflict between men and microbes are what strike the mind. What is less readily apprehended is the more common fact that infection can occur without producing disease.[4]

The principal evidence that the vaccines are effective actually dates from the more recent period, during which time the dreaded polio epidemics of the 1940s and 1950s have never reappeared in the developed countries, and measles, mumps, and rubella, which even a generation ago were among the commonest diseases of childhood, have become far less prevalent, at least in their classic acute forms, since the triple MMR vaccine was introduced into common use.

Yet how the vaccines actually accomplish these changes is not nearly as well understood as most people like to think it is. The disturbing possibility that they act in some other way than by producing a genuine immunity is suggested by the fact that the diseases in question have continued to break out even in highly immunized populations, and that in such cases the observed differences in incidence and severity between immunized and unimmunized persons have tended to be far less dramatic than expected, and in some cases not measurably significant at all.

In a recent British outbreak of whooping cough, for example, even fully immunized children contracted the disease in fairly large numbers, and the rates of serious complications and death were reduced only slightly.[5] In another recent outbreak of pertussis, 46 of the 85 fully immunized children studied eventually contracted the disease.[6]

In 1977, 344 new cases of measles were reported on the campus of UCLA in a population that was supposedly 91 percent immune, according to careful serological testing.[7] Another 20 cases of measles were reported in the Pecos, New Mexico, area within a period of a few months in 1981, and 75 percent of them had been fully immunized, some of them quite recently.[8] A survey of sixth-graders in a well-immunized urban community revealed that about 15 percent of this age group are still susceptible to rubella, a figure essentially identical with that of the prevaccine era.[9]

Finally, although the overall incidence of typical acute measles in the U.S. has dropped sharply from about 400,000 cases annually in the early 1960s to about 30,000 cases by 1974–76, the death rate remained exactly the same;[10] and, with the peak incidence now occurring in adolescents and young adults, the risk of pneumonia and demonstrable liver abnormalities has actually increased substantially, according to one recent study, to well over 3 percent and 20 percent, respectively.[11]

The simplest way to explain these discrepancies would be to postulate that the vaccines confer only partial or temporary immunity, which sounds reasonable enough given the fact that they are either live viruses rendered less virulent by serial passage in tissue culture, or bacteria or bacterial proteins that have been killed or denatured by heat, such that they can still elicit an antibody response but no longer initiate the full-blown disease.

Because the vaccine is a "trick," in the sense that it simulates the true or natural immune response developed in the course of recovering from the actual disease, it is certainly realistic to expect that such artificial immunity will in fact "wear off" quite easily, and even require additional "booster" doses at regular intervals throughout life to maintain peak effectiveness.

Such an explanation would be disturbing enough for most people. Indeed, the basic fallacy inherent in it is painfully evident in the fact that there is no way to know how long this partial or temporary immunity will last in any given individual, or how often it will need to be restimulated, because the answers to these questions clearly depend on precisely the same individual variables that would have determined whether or how severely the same person, unvaccinated, would have contracted the disease in the first place.

In any case, a number of other observations suggests equally strongly that this simple explanation cannot be the correct one. In the first place, a number of investigators have shown that when a person vaccinated against the measles, for example, again becomes susceptible to it, even repeated booster doses will have little or no effect.[12]

In the second place, the vaccines do not act merely by producing pale or mild copies of the original disease; all of them also commonly produce a variety of symptoms of their own. Moreoever, in some cases, these illnesses may be considerably more serious than the original disease, involving deeper structures, more vital organs, and less of a tendency to resolve spontaneously. Even more worrisome is the fact that they are almost always more difficult to recognize.

Thus, in a recent outbreak of mumps in supposedly immune school-children, several developed atypical symptoms, such as anorexia, vomiting, and erythematous rashes, without any parotid involvement, and the diagnosis required extensive serological testing to rule out other concurrent disease.[13] The syndrome of "atypical measles" can be equally difficult to diagnose, even when it is thought of,[14] which suggests that is is often overlooked entirely. In some cases, atypical measles can be much more severe than the regular kind, with pneumonia, petechiae, edema, and severe pain,[15] and likewise can often go unsuspected.

In any case, it seems virtually certain that other vaccine-related syndromes will be described and identified, if only we take the trouble to look for them, and that the ones we are aware of so far represent only a very small part of the problem. But even these few make it less and less plausible to assume that the vaccines produce a normal, healthy immunity that lasts for some time but then *wears off*, leaving the patient miraculously unharmed and unaffected by the experience.

2. Some Personal Experiences with Vaccine-Related Illness

I would like now to present a few of my own vaccine cases, both to give a sense of their variety and chronicity, and to show how difficult it can be to trace them, and also to begin to address the crucial question that is too seldom even asked, namely, how the vaccines actually *work*, i.e., what effects they do in fact produce in the human body.

My first case was that of an eight-month-old girl with recurrent fevers of unknown origin. I first saw her in January of 1977, a few weeks after her third such episode. These were brief, lasting 48 hours at most, but very intense, with the fever typically reaching 105°F. During the second episode, she was hospitalized for diagnostic evaluation, but her pediatrician found nothing out of the ordinary. Apart from these episodes, the child felt quite well, and appeared to be growing and developing normally.

I could get no further information from the mother, except for the fact that the episodes had occurred almost exactly one month apart; and, upon consulting her calendar, we learned that the first episode had come exactly one month after the last of her DPT injections, which had also been given at monthly intervals. At this point, the mother remembered that the child had had similar febrile episodes immediately after each injection, but that she had been instructed to ignore them, inasmuch as they are "common reactions" to the vaccine. I therefore gave the child a single *oral* dose of dilute homeopathic DPT vaccine; and I am happy to report that the child has remained well since, with no further episodes of any kind.

This case illustrates how homeopathic remedies prepared from vaccines can be used for *diagnosis* as well as treatment of vaccine-related illnesses, which, no matter how strongly they are suspected, might otherwise be almost impossible to substantiate.

Secondly, because fever is the commonest known complication of the pertussis vaccine, and inasmuch as the child seemed quite well between the attacks, her response to the vaccine appeared to be a relatively strong and healthy one, disturbing because of its recurrence and periodicity, but in any case relatively simple to cure, as indeed it proved to be. But one cannot help wondering what happens to the vaccine in those tens of millions of children who show no obvious reponse to it at all.

Since that time, I have seen numerous cases of children with recurrent fevers of unknown origin, associated with a variety of other chronic complaints, chiefly irritability, temper tantrums, and increased susceptibility to colds, tonsillitis, and ear infections, which were similarly traceable to the pertussis vaccine, and which responded successfully to treatment with the homeopathic DPT nosode. Indeed, I would have to say, on the basis of that experience, that the DPT vaccine is probably one of the major causes of recurrent fevers of unknown origin in small children today.

My second case was that of a 9½-month-old girl, who presented acutely with a fever of 105° F., and very few other symptoms. Like the first, this child had had two similar episodes previously, but at irregular intervals; and the parents, who felt ambivalent about vaccinations in general, had given her only one dose of the DPT vaccine so far, although the first episode occurred a few weeks afterwards.

I first saw the child in June of 1978. The fever remained high and unremitting for 48 hours, despite the usual acute remedies and supportive measures. A CBC revealed a white count of 32,100 per mm.3, with 43 percent lymphocytes, 11 percent monocytes, 25 percent neutrophilis (many with toxic granulations), and 1 percent metamyelocytes and other immature forms. When I asked a pediatrician about these findings, "pertussis" was his immediate reply. After a single oral dose of homeopathic DPT vaccine, the fever came down abruptly within a few hours, and the child has remained well since.

This case was disturbing mainly because of the hematological abnormalities, which were in the leukemoid range, together with the absence of any cough or distinctive respiratory symptoms, which suggested that introducing the vaccine directly into the blood may actually promote deeper or more systematic pathology than allowing the pertussis organism to set up typical symptoms of local inflammation at the normal portal of entry.

The third case was a five-year-old boy with chronic lymphocytic leukemia, whom I happened to see in August of 1978, while visiting an old friend and teacher, a family physician with over 40 years' experience. Well out of earshot of either the boy or his parents, he told me that the leukemia had first appeared following a DPT vaccination, and that, although he had treated the child successfully with natural remedies on two previous occasions, with shrinking of the liver and spleen to approximately normal size, and dramatic improvement in the blood picture, full relapse had occurred soon after each successive DPT booster.

The idea that vaccinations might also be implicated in some cases of childhood leukemia was shocking enough in itself, but it also completed the line of reasoning opened up by the previous case. For leukemia is a cancerous process of the blood and the blood-forming organs, the liver, the spleen, the lymph nodes, and the bone marrow, which are also the basic anatomical units of the immune system. Insofar as the vaccines are capable of producing serious complications at all, the blood and the immune organs would certainly be the logical place to begin looking for them.

But perhaps even more shocking to me is the fact that the boy's own physician dared not communicate his suspicion of vaccine-related illness to the parents, let alone to the general public. It was this case that convinced me, once and for all, of the need for serious, public discussion of our collected experiences with vaccine-related illness, precisely because rigorous experimental proof will require years of investigation and a firm public commitment that has not even been made yet.

I will now present two cases from my limited experience with MMR vaccine.

In December of 1980 I saw a three-year-old boy with a four-week history of loss of appetite, stomachaches, indigestion, and swollen glands. The stomach pains were quite severe, and often accompanied by belching, flatulence, and explosive diarrhea. The nose was also congested, and the lower eyelids were quite red. The mother also reported some unusual behavior changes, such as extreme untidiness, "wild" and "noisy" playing, and waking at 2 A.M. to get into bed with the parents.

The physical examination was unremarkable except for some large, tender left posterior auricular and suboccipital nodes, and marked enlargement of the tonsils. I then learned that the child had received the MMR vaccine in October, about two weeks before the onset of symptoms, with no apparent reaction to it at the time. I gave the child a single dose of the homeopathic rubella vaccine, and the symptoms promptly disappeared within 48 hours.

In April 1981, the parents brought him back for a slight fever, and another three-week history of intermittent pain in and behind the right ear, stuffy nose, etc. On examination, the whole right side of the face appeared to be swollen, especially the cheek and the angle of the jaw. The right eye was red and infected. He responded well to acute homeopathic remedies and has remained well since.

This boy was typical of my rubella vaccine cases. At an interval of a few weeks after the MMR vaccine, which is about the same as the normal incubation period of rubella, a rather nondescript illness develops, which becomes subacute and rather more severe than rubella in the same age group, with, e.g., abdominal or joint pains and marked adenopathy, but no rash. Usually the diagnosis is suspected because of the characteristic posterior auricular and suboccipital nodes, and confirmed by a favorable response to the homeopathic rubella nosode.

As I read over this case, I am struck by the possibility that his second illness, and especially the parotid enlargement, may have represented continuing activity of the mumps component of the vaccine, inasmuch as I did not have the triple MMR nosode, but only those derived from the individual components. We must therefore also consider the probability that a variety of "mixed" or composite syndromes may occur, representing the patient's responses to two or all three of the vaccine components, either simultaneously or over time.

In April of 1981 I first saw a four-year-old boy for bilateral chronic enlargement of the posterior auricular nodes, which were also occasionally tender. The mother had noticed the swelling for about one year, during which time he had become more susceptible to various upper respiratory infections, none of them especially severe. The mother had also noticed recurrent parotid swelling at irregular intervals over the same time period, which began shortly after the MMR vaccine was given at the age of three.

At the time of the first visit, the child was not ill, and because the mother was about two months pregnant at the time, I elected to observe the child and do nothing if possible until the pregnancy was over. He did develop a mild laryngitis in the last trimester, which responded well to bed rest and simple homeopathic remedies.

In April of 1982, he came down with acute bronchitis. I noticed that the posterior auricular nodes were once again swollen and tender and decided to give him the homoeopathic rubella nosode at that point. The cough promptly subsided, and the nodes regressed in size and were no longer tender. Two weeks later, however, he returned with a noticeably hard, tender swelling on the outside of the right cheek, near the angle of the jaw, and some pain on chewing or opening the mouth. A single dose of the homeopathic mumps nosode was given, and the child has been well since.

In this case also, we see the subacute pattern of the disease, with a strong tendency to chronicity and increased susceptibility to weaker, low-grade responses, in contrast to the vigorous, acute responses typically associated with diseases like the measles and the mumps when acquired naturally.

3. How Do the Vaccines Work?

It is dangerously misleading, and, indeed, the exact opposite of the truth to claim that a vaccine makes us "immune" or *protects* us against an acute disease, if in fact it only drives the disease deeper into the interior and causes us to harbor it *chronically*, with the result that our responses to it become progressively weaker, and show less and less tendency to heal or resolve themselves spontaneously.

What I propose, then, is simply to investigate as thoroughly and objectively as we can how the vaccines actually *work* inside the human body, and to begin by paying attention to the implications of what we already know. In particular, I would like to consider in detail the process of falling ill with and recovering from a typical acute disease, such as the measles, in contrast with what we can observe following the administration of the measles vaccine.

We all know that measles is primarily a virus of the respiratory tract, both because it is inhaled by susceptible persons upon contact with infected droplets in the air, and because these droplets are produced by the coughing and sneezing of a person with the disease.

Once inhaled by a susceptible person, the measles virus then undergoes a long period of silent multiplication, first in the tonsils, adenoids, and accessory lymphoid tissues of the nasopharynx; later in the regional lymph nodes of the head and neck; and, eventually, several days later, it passes into the blood and enters the spleen, the liver, the thymus, and the bone marrow, the visceral organs of the immune system.[16] Throughout this incubation period, which lasts from 10 to 14 days, the patient usually feels quite well and experiences few or no symptoms.[17]

By the time that the first symptoms of measles appear, circulating antibodies are already detectable in the blood, and the height of the symptomatology coincides with the peak of the antibody response.[18] In other words, the "illness" is simply the definitive effort of the immune system to clear the virus from the blood. Equally noteworthy is the fact that the virus is eliminated by sneezing and coughing, i.e., via the same route through which it entered in the first place.

It is evident that the process of *mounting* an acute illness like the measles, no less than recovering from it, involves a general mobilization of the entire immune system, including inflammation of the previously sensitized tissues at the portal of entry, activation of leukocytes and macrophages, liberation of the serum complement system, and a host of other mechanisms, of which the production of circulating antibody is only one, and by no means the most important.

Such a splendid outpouring leaves little doubt that such illnesses are in fact the decisive experiences in the normal physiological maturation of the immune system as a whole in the life of a healthy child. For not only will the child who recovers from the measles never again be susceptible to it;[19] such an experience also cannot fail to prepare the individual to respond even more promptly and effectively to any infections he may acquire in the future. The ability to mount a vigorous acute response to organisms of this type must therefore be reckoned among the most fundamental requirements of general health and well-being.

In contrast, when an artificially attenuated virus such as measles is injected directly into the blood, bypassing the normal portal of entry, at most a brief inflammatory reaction may be noted at the injection site, or in the regional lymph nodes; but there is no "incubation period" of local contact at the normal portal of entry, and consequently very little possibility of eliminating the virus via the same route.

Even more important is the fact that the virus has been artificially "attenuated," so that it will no longer initiate a generalized inflammatory response, or indeed any of the nonspecific defense mechanisms that help us to respond to infection generally. By "tricking" the body in this fashion, we have accomplished what the entire immune system seems to have evolved in order to prevent: We have placed the virus directly into the blood, and given it free and immediate access to the major immune organs, without any obvious way of getting rid of it.

The result is, indeed, the production of circulating antibodies against the virus; but the antibody response now occurs as an isolated technical feat, without any generalized inflammatory response, or any noticeable improvement in the general health of the organism. Exactly the opposite, in fact: The price that we have to pay for those antibodies is the persistence of virus elements in the blood for prolonged periods of time, perhaps permanently, which in turn presupposes a systematic weakening of our ability to mount an effective response not only to measles, but also to other acute infections as well.

Far from producing a genuine immunity, then, the vaccines may act by actually interfering with or *suppressing* the immune response as a whole, in much the same way that radiation, chemotherapy, and corticosteroids and other anti-inflammatory drugs do. Artificial immunization focuses on *antibody production*, a single aspect of the immune process, and disarticulates it and allows it to stand for the whole, in much the same way as chemical suppression of an elevated blood pressure is accepted as a valid substitute for a genuine *cure* of the patient whose blood pressure has risen. Worst of all, by making it difficult or impossible to mount a vigorous, acute response to infection, artificial immunization substitutes for it a much weaker, *chronic* response with little or no tendency to heal itself spontaneously.

Moreover, adequate models already exist for predicting and explaining what sorts of chronic disease are likely to result from the chronic, long-term persistence of viruses and other foreign proteins within the cells of the immune system. It has long been known that live viruses, for example, are capable of surviving or remaining latent within the host cells for years, without continually provoking acute disease. They do so simply by attaching their own genetic material as an extra particle or "episome" to the genome of the host cell, and replicating along with it, which allows the host cell to continue its own normal funtions for the most part, but imposes on it additional instructions for the synthesis of viral proteins.[20]

Latent viruses of this type have already been implicated in three distinct types of chronic disease, namely (1) *recurrent or episodic acute diseases* such as herpes, shingles, warts, etc.[21]; (2) *"slow-virus" diseases*, i.e., subacute or chronic, progressive, often fatal conditions, such as kuru, Creutzfeldt-Jakob disease, subacute sclerosing panencephalitis (SSPE), AIDS, and possibly Guillain-Barre syndrome[22]; and (3) *tumors*, both benign and malignant.[23]

In any case, the latent virus survives as a clearly "foreign" element within the cell, which means that the immune system must continue to try to make antibodies against it, insofar as it can still respond to it at all. Because the virus is now permanently incorporated within the genetic material of the cell, these antibodies will now have to be directed against the cell itself.

The persistence of live viruses or other foreign antigens within the cells of the host therefore cannot fail to provoke *auto-immune* pheno-mena, because destroying the infected cells is now the only possible way that this constant antigenic challenge can be removed from the body. Since routine vaccination introduces live viruses and other highly antigenic material into the blood of virtually every living person, it is difficult to escape the conclusion that a significant harvest of auto-immune diseases will automatically result.

Sir Macfarlane Burnet has observed that the components of the immune system all function as if they were collectively designed to help the organism to discriminate "self" from "nonself," i.e., to help us to recognize and tolerate our own cells, and to identify and eliminate foreign or extraneous substances as completely as possible.[24] This concept is exemplified not only by the acute response to infection, but also by the rejection of transplanted tissues, or "homografts," both of which result in the complete and permanent removal of the offending substance from the body.

If Burnet is correct, then latent viruses, auto-immune phenomena, and cancer would seem to represent different aspects of the same basic dilemma, which the immune system can neither escape nor resolve. For all of them presuppose a certain degree of *chronic immune failure,* a state in which it becomes difficult or impossible for the body either to recognize its own cells as unambiguously its own, or to eliminate its parasites as unequivocally foreign.

In the case of the attenuated measles virus, it is not difficult to imagine that introducing it directly into the blood would continue to provoke an antibody response for a considerable period of time, which is doubtless the whole point of giving the vaccine; but that eventually, as the virus succeeded in attaining a state of latency within the cell, the antibody response would wane, both because circulating antibodies cannot normally cross the cell membrane, and also because they are powerful immunosuppressive agents in their own right.[25]

The effect of circulating antibody will thereafter be mainly to keep the virus *within* the cell, i.e., to continue to prevent any acute inflammatory response, until eventually, perhaps under circumstances of accumulated stress or emergency, this precarious balance breaks down, antibodies begin to be produced in large quantities against the cells themselves, and frank auto-immune phenomena of necrosis and tissue destruction supervene. Latent viruses, in this sense, are like biological "time bombs," set to explode at an indeterminate time in the future.[26]

Auto-immune diseases have always seemed obscure, aberrant, and bizarre, because it is not intuitively obvious why the body should suddenly begin to attack and destroy its own tissues. They make a lot more sense, and, indeed, must be reckoned as "healthy," if destroying the chronically infected cells is the only possible way of eliminating an even more serious threat to life, namely, the persistence of the foreign antigenic challenge within the cells of the host.

Tumor formation could then be understood as simply a more advanced stage of chronic immune failure, according to the same model. For, as long as the host is subjected to enormous and unremitting pressure to make antibodies against itself, that response will automatically tend to become less and less effective.

Eventually, under stress of this magnitude, the auto-immune mechanism could easily break down to the point that the chronically infected and genetically transformed cells, no longer clearly "self" or "nonself," begin to free themselves from the normal restraints of "histocompatibility" within the architecture of the surrounding cells, and begin to multiply autonomously at their expense.

A tumor could then be described as "benign" insofar as the breakdown of histocompatibility remains strictly localized to the tissue of origin, and "malignant" insofar as it begins to spread to other cell types, tissues, and organs, even in more remote areas. Malignancy might simply represent the reactivation of the virus from its latent phase into a more acute mode, albeit with less inflammation and more tissue destruction than the original wild-type infection.

If what I am saying turns out to be true, then what we have done by artificial immunizations is essentially to trade off our acute, epidemic disease of the past century for the weaker and far less curable chronic diseases of the present, with their amortizable suffering and disability. In doing so, we have also opened up limitless evolutionary possibilities for the future of ongoing *in vivo* genetic recombination within the cells of the race.

4. The Individual Vaccines Reconsidered

I want next to consider each of the vaccines on an individual basis, in relation to the infectious diseases from which they are derived.

The MMR is composed of attenuated live measles, mumps, and rubella viruses administered in a single intramuscular injection at about 15 months of age. Subsequent reimmunization is no longer recommended, except for young women of childbearing age, in whom the risk of congenital rubella syndrome (CRS) is thought to warrant it, even though the effectiveness of reimmunization is questionable at best.

Prior to the vaccine era, measles, mumps, and rubella were reckoned among the "routine childhood diseases," which most schoolchildren contracted before the age of puberty, and from which nearly all recovered with permanent, lifelong immunity, and no complications or sequelae.

But they were not always so harmless. Measles, in particular, can be a devastating disease when a population encounters it for the first time. Its importation from Spain, for instance, undoubtedly contributed to Cortez' conquest of the great Aztec Empire: Whole villages were carried off by epidemics of measles and smallpox, leaving only a small remnant of cowed, superstitious warriors to face the bearded *conquistadores* from across the sea.[27] In more recent outbreaks among isolated, primitive people, the case fatality rate from measles averaged 20 to 30 percent.[28]

In these so-called "virgin-soil" epidemics, not only measles but also polio and many other similar diseases take their highest toll of death and serious complications among adolescents and young adults, healthy and vigorous people in the prime of life, and leave relatively unharmed the group of school-age children before the age of puberty.[29]

This means that the evolution of a disease such as measles from a dreaded killer to an ordinary disease of childhood presupposes the development of nonspecific or "herd" immunity in young children, such that, when they are finally exposed to the disease, it activates defense mechanisms already prepared and in place, resulting in the long incubation period and the usually benign, self-limited course described above.

Under these circumstances, the rationale for wanting to vaccinate young children against measles is limited to the fact that a very small number of deaths and serious complications have continued to occur, chiefly pneumonia, encephalitis, and the rare but dreaded subacute sclerosing panencephalitis (SSPE), a slow-virus disease with a reported incidence of 1 per 100,000 cases.[30] Pneumonia, by far the commonest complication, is usually benign and self-limited, even without treatment[31]; and, even in those rare cases in which bacterial pneumonia supervenes, adequate treatment is currently available.

By all accounts, then, the death rate from wild-type measles is very low, the incidence of serious sequelae is insignificant, and the general benefit to the child who recovers from the disease, and to his contacts and descendants, is very great. Consequently, even if the measles vaccine could be shown to reduce the risk of death or serious complications from the disease, it still could not justify the high probability of auto-immune diseases, cancer, and whatever else may result from the propagation of latent measles virus in human tissue culture for life.

Ironically, what the measles vaccine certainly has done is to reverse the historical or evolutionary process to the extent that measles is once again a disease of adolescents and young adults,[32] with a correspondingly higher incidence of pneumonia and other complications and a general tendency to be a more serious and disabling disease than it usually is in younger children.

As for the claim that the vaccine has helped to eliminate measles encephalitis, I myself, in my own relatively small general practice, have already seen two children with major seizure disorders which the parents clearly ascribed to the measles vaccine, although they would never have been able to prove the connection in a court of law, and never considered the possibility of compensation.

Such cases therefore never make the official statistics, and are accordingly omitted from conventional surveys of the problem. Merely injecting the virus into the blood would naturally favor a higher incidence of deep or visceral complications affecting the lungs, liver, and brain, for which the measles virus has a known affinity.

The case for immunizing against mumps and rubella seems *a fortiori* even more tenuous, for exactly the same reasons. Mumps is also essentially a benign, self-limited disease in children before the age of puberty, and recovery from a single attack confers lifelong immunity. The principal complication is meningoencephalitis, mild or subclinical forms of which are relatively common, although the death rate is extremely low,[33] and sequelae are rare.

The mumps vaccine is prepared and administered in much the same way as the measles, usually in the same injection; and the dangers associated with it are likewise comparable. Again, like the measles, mumps is fast becoming a disease of adolescents and young adults,[34] age groups which do not tolerate the disease as well. The chief complication is acute epididymo-orchitis, which occurs in 30 to 40 percent of the males affected past the age of puberty, and usually results in atrophy of the testicle on the affected side[35]; but it also shows a strong tendency to attack the ovary and the pancreas.

For all of these reasons, the greatest favor we could do for our children would be to expose them all to the measles and mumps when they are young, which would not only protect them against contracting more serious forms of these diseases when they grow older, but would also greatly assist in their immunological maturation with minimal risk. I need hardly add that this is very close to the actual evolution of these diseases before the MMR vaccine was introduced.

The same discrepancy is evident in the case of rubella, or "German measles," which in young children is a disease so mild that it frequently escapes detection,[36] but in older children and adults not infrequently produces arthritis, purpura, and other severe, systemic signs.[37] The main impetus for the development of the vaccine was certainly the recognition of the congenital rubella syndrome (CRS) resulting from damage to the developing embryo in utero during the first trimester of pregnancy,[38] and the relatively high incidence of CRS traceable to the rubella outbreak of 1964.

But here again, we have an almost entirely benign, self-limited disease transformed by the vaccine into a considerably less benign disease of adolescents and young adults of reproductive age, which is, ironically, the group that most needs to be protected against it. Moreover, as with measles and mumps, the simplest and most effective way to prevent CRS would be to expose everybody to rubella in elementary school; re-infection does sometimes occur after recovery from rubella, but much less commonly than after vaccination.[39]

The equation looks somewhat different for the diphtheria and tetanus vaccines. First of all, both diphtheria and tetanus are serious, sometimes fatal diseases, even under the best of treament; this is especially true of tetanus, which still carries a mortality of anywhere from 20 to 50 percent.

Furthermore, these vaccines are not made from living diphtheria and tetanus organisms, but only from certain "toxins" elaborated by them; these poisonous substances are still highly antigenic, even after being inactivated by heat. Diphtheria and tetanus "toxoids" therefore do not protect against infection per se, but only against the systemic action of the original poisons in the absence of which both infections are of minor importance clinically.

Consequently, it is easy to understand why parents might want their children protected against diphtheria and tetanus, if safe and effective protection were available. Moreover, both vaccines have been in use for a long time, and the reported incidence of serious problems has remained very low, so that there has never been much public outcry against them.

On the other hand, both diseases are quite readily controlled by simple sanitary measures and careful attention to wound hygiene; and, in any case, both have been steadily disappearing from the developing countries, since long before the vaccines were introduced.

Diphtheria now occurs sporadically in the United States, often in areas with significant reservoirs of unvaccinated children. But the claim that the vaccine is "protective" is once again belied by the fact that, when the disease does break out, the supposedly "susceptible" children are in fact no more likely to develop clinical diphtheria than their fully immunized contacts. In a 1969 outbreak in Chicago, for example, the Board of Health reported that 25 percent of the cases had been fully immunized and that another 12 percent had received one or more doses of the vaccine and showed serological evidence of full immunity; another 18 percent had been partly immunized according to the same criteria.[40]

So, once again, we are faced with the probability that what the diphtheria toxoid has produced is not a genuine immunity to diphtheria at all, but rather some sort of chronic immune *tolerance* to it, by harboring highly antigenic residues somewhere within the cells of the immune system, presumably with long-term suppressive effects on the immune mechanism generally.

This suspicion is further aggravated by the fact that all of the DPT vaccines are alum-precipitated and preserved with thimerosal, an organomercury derivative, to prevent them from being metabolized too rapidly, so that the antigenic challenge will continue for as long as possible. The fact is that we do not know and have never even attempted to discover what actually becomes of these foreign substances once they are inside the human body.

Exactly the same problems complicate the record of the tetanus vaccine, which almost certainly has had at least some impact in reducing the incidence of tetanus in its classic acute form, yet presumably also survives for years or even decades as a potent foreign antigen within the body, with long-term effects on the immune system and elsewhere that are literally incalculable.

"Whooping cough," much like diphtheria and tetanus, began to decline as a serious epidemiological threat long before the vaccine was introduced. Moreover, the vaccine has not been particularly effective, even according to its proponents; and the incidence of known side effects is disturbingly high.

The power of the pertussis vaccine to damage the central nervous system, for example, has received growing attention since Stewart and his colleagues reported an alarmingly high incidence of encephalopathy and severe convulsive disorders in British children that were traceable to the vaccine.[41] My own cases, a few of which were reported above, suggest that hematological disturbances may be even more prevalent, and that, in any case, the *known* complications almost certainly represent a small fraction of the total.

In any case, the pertussis vaccine has become controversial even in the United States, where medical opinion has remained almost unanimously in favor of immunizations generally; and several countries, such as West Germany, have discontinued routine pertussis vaccination entirely.[42]

Pertussis is also extremely variable clinically, ranging in severity from asymptomatic, mild, or inapparent infections, which are quite common actually, to very rare cases in young infants less than five months of age, in which the mortality is said to reach 40 percent.[43] Indeed, the disease is rarely fatal or even that serious in children over a year old, and antibiotics have very little to do with the outcome.[44]

A good deal of the pressure to immunize at the present time thus seems to be attributable to the higher death rate in very young infants, which has led to the terrifying practice of giving this most clearly dangerous of the vaccines to infants at two months of age, when their mother's milk would normally have protected them from all infections about as well as it can ever be done,[45] and the effect on the still developing blood and nervous system could be catastrophic.

For all of these reasons, the practice of routine pertussis immunization should be discontinued as quickly as possible and more studies done to assess and compensate the damage that it has already done.

Poliomyelitis and the polio vaccines present an entirely different situation. The standard Sabin vaccine is trivalent, consisting of attenuated, live polioviruses of each of the three strains associated with poliomyelitis; but it is administered orally, in much the same way as the infection is acquired in nature. The oral or noninjectable route, which leaves the recipient free to develop a natural immunity at the normal portal of entry, i.e., the GI tract, would therefore appear to represent a considerable safety factor.

On the other hand, the wild-type poliovirus produces no symptoms whatsoever in over 90 percent of the people who contact it, even under epidemic conditions[46]; and, of those people who do come down with recognizable clinical disease, perhaps only 1 or 2 percent ever progress to the full-blown neurological picture of "poliomyelitis," with its characteristic lesions in the anterior horn cells of the spinal cord or medulla oblongata.[47]

Poliomyelitis thus presupposes peculiar conditions of susceptibility in the host, even a specific *anatomical* susceptibility, since, even under epidemic conditions, the virulence of the poliovirus is so low, and the number of cases resulting in death or permanent disability was always remarkably small.[48]

Given the fact that the poliovirus was ubiquitous before the vaccine was introduced, and could be found routinely in samples of city sewage wherever it was looked for,[49] it is evident that effective, natural immunity to poliovirus was already as close to being universal as it can ever be, and a fortiori that no artificial substitute could ever equal or even approximate that result. Indeed, because the virulence of the poliovirus was so low to begin with, it is difficult to see what further attenuation of it could possibly accomplish, other than to abate as well the full vigor of the natural immune response to it.

For the fact remains that even the attenuated virus is still alive, and that the people who were anatomically susceptible to it before are still susceptible to it now. This means, of course, that at least *some* of these same people will develop paralytic polio from the vaccine,[50] and that the others may still be harboring the virus in latent form, perhaps within those same cells.

The only obvious advantage of giving the vaccine, then, would be to introduce the population to the virus when they are still infants, and the virulence is normally lowest anyway[51]; and even this benefit could be more than offset by the danger of weakening the immune response, as we have seen. In any case, the whole matter is clearly one of enormous complexity, and illustrates only too well the hidden dangers and miscalculations that are inherent in the virtually irresistible attempt to beat nature at her own game, to eliminate a problem that cannot be eliminated, i.e., the susceptibility to disease itself.

So even in the case of the polio vaccine, which appears to be about as safe as any vaccine ever *can* be, the same fundamental dilemma remains. Perhaps the day will come when we can face the consequences of deliberately feeding live polioviruses to every living infant, and admit that we should have left well enough alone, and addressed ourselves to the art of healing the sick when we have to, rather than to the technology of eradicating the *possibility* of sickness, when we don't have to, and can't possibly succeed in any case.

5. Vaccination and the Path of Medical Technology

In conclusion, I want to go back to the beginning, to the essentially political aspects of vaccination, that oblige us all to reason and deliberate together about matters of common concern, and to reach a clear decision about how we choose to live. I have stated my own views regarding the safety and effectiveness of the vaccines, and I hope that others of differing views will do the same.

That is why I am deeply troubled by the atmosphere of fanaticism with which the vaccines are imposed on the public, and serious discussion of them is ignored or stifled by the medical authorities, as if the question had already been settled definitively and for all time. In the words of Sir Macfarlane Burnet:

> It is our pride that in a civilized country the only infectious diseases which anyone is likely to suffer are either trivial or easily cured by available drugs. The diseases that killed in the past have in one way or another been rendered impotent, and, in the process, general principles of control have been developed which should be applicable to any unexpected outbreak in the future.[52]

Quite apart from the truth of these claims, they exemplify the smugness and self-righteousness of a profession and a society that worships its own ability to manipulate and control the processes of nature itself. That is why, as Robert Mendelsohn has said, "We are quick to pull the trigger, but slow to examine the consequences of our actions."[53]

Indeed, one would have to say, *methodically* slow. In 1978, for example, the American Academy of Pediatrics, which had been charged by Congress with responsibility to formulate guidelines for federal compensation of "vaccination-related injuries," issued the following eligibility restrictions:

> 1. Compensation should be made available to any child or young person under the age of 18 years, or a contact of such person of any age, who suffers a major reaction to a vaccine mandated for school entry or continuation in his or her state of residence.
>
> 2. Such a reaction should have been previously recognized as a possible consequence of the vaccine given.
>
> 3. Such a reaction should have occurred no more than 30 days following the immunization.[54]

These restrictions would automatically exclude all of the chronic diseases, or indeed anything other than the very few adverse reactions that have so far been identified, which clearly represent only a tiny fraction of the problem.

Still less can either the government or the medical establishment be considered ignorant of the possibility that lurks in every parent's mind and heart, namely, that the vaccines cause cancer and other chronic diseases. Precisely that possibility was raised by Professor Robert Simpson of Rutgers in a 1976 seminar for science writers sponsored by the American Cancer Society:

> Immunization programs against flu, measles, mumps, polio, and so forth, may actually be seeding humans with RNA to form latent proviruses in cells throughout the body. These latent proviruses could be molecules in search of diseases; when activated, under proper conditions, they could cause a variety of diseases, including rheumatoid arthritis, multiple sclerosis, systemic lupus erythematosus, Parkinson's disease, and perhaps cancer.[55]

Unfortunately, this is the sort of warning that very few pe
willing or able to hear at this point, least of all the American Cancer
Society or the American Academy of Pediatrics. The fact is, as Dubos
points out, that all of us still want to believe in the "miracle," regardless
of the evidence:

> The faith in the magical power of drugs often blunts the critical senses,
> and comes close at times to a mass hysteria, involving scientists and laymen
> alike. Men want miracles as much today as in the past. If they do not join
> one of the newer cults, they satisfy this need by worshipping at the altar of
> modern science. This faith in the magical power of drugs is not new. It
> helped to give medicine the authority of a priesthood and to recreate the
> glamour of ancient mysteries.[56]

The idea of eradicating measles or polio has come to seem attractive to
us simply because the power of medical science makes it seem technically
possible; we worship every victory of technology over nature, just as the
bullfight celebrates the truimph of human intelligence over the brute
beast.

That is why we do not begrudge the drug companies their enormous
profits, and gladly volunteer our own bodies and those of our children
for their latest experiments. Vaccination is essentially a religious sacrament of our own participation in the miracle, a veritable auto-da-fe in the
name of modern civilization itself.

Nobody in his right mind would seriously entertain the idea that if we
could somehow eliminate, one by one, measles and polio and all the
known diseases of mankind, we would be any the healthier for it, or that
other even more serious diseases would not quickly take their places.

Still less would a rational being suppose that the illnesses from which
he suffered were "entities" somehow separable from the patients who
suffer them, and that, with the appropriate chemical or surgical sacrament, this separation can literally be carried out.

Yet these are precisely the "miracles" we are taught to believe in, and
the idolatries to which we aspire. We prefer to forget the older and
simpler truths, that the propensity or susceptibility to illness is deeply
rooted in our biological nature and that the phenomena of disease are the
expression of our own life energy, trying to overcome whatever it is
trying to overcome, trying, in short to *heal itself.*

The myth that we can find technical solutions for all human ailments
seems attractive at first, precisely because it bypasses the problem of

healing, which is a genuine miracle in the sense that it can always *fail* to occur. We are all genuinely at risk of illness and death at every moment; no amount of technology can change that. Yet the mission of technical medicine is precisely to try to change that: to stand at all times in the front lines against disease, and to attack and destroy it whenever and wherever it shows itself.

That is why, with all due respect, I cannot have faith in the miracles or accept the sacraments of Merck, Sharp, and Dohme and the Center for Disease Control. I prefer to stay with the miracle of life itself, which has given us illness and disease, but also the arts of medicine and healing, through which we can acknowledge and experience our pain and our vulnerability, and sometimes, with the grace of God and the help of our fellow men, an awareness of health and well-being that transcends all boundaries. That is *my* religion; and, while I would willingly share it, I would not *force* it on anyone.

Postscript on Immunizations: Directions for Future Research

In "Immunizations—A Dissenting View," my intention was simply to understand my own experience, to develop a coherent and plausible line of reasoning that could explain what I had read and felt and thought about, and what my patients were telling me.

The next step is to address the issue of *experimental verification*, to try to sketch out where and how we might look for valid, repeatable evidence for the efficacy, safety, and mode of action of the common vaccines.

As I reread the argument, I realized that even the more speculative ideas in it could in fact be tested quite easily with the standard research techniques now in common use. Because I myself have very little research training or experience, I am doubly curious why such tests were not carried out long ago.

A number of scholars have certainly *entertained* these ideas before, as I indicated in the text, and even considered them publicly. The only obstacle that I can see to taking them seriously is that they are "heretical," that it would be impossible even to take the time to study them without a "paradigm shift" of some magnitude.[57]

1. How Effective Are the Vaccines?

If the vaccines act by *suppressing* the ability of the organism to mount an effective acute inflammatory response, then we can no longer accept a simple drop in the incidence of the acute disease as a measure of true immunity. I also argued that the mere presence of circulating antibody cannot suffice either, because the diseases in question do continue to break out, even in serologically highly "immune" populations.

What strikes me as a far more interesting and relevant measurement is the degree to which the vaccine "protects" against the acute disease when the latter actually does break out. This could be determined relatively easily by studying the incidence and morbidity of each disease in fully and partly immunized populations, as compared with those of their nonimmunized neighbors. Such a study would still have nothing to say about the possibility of immunosuppression. But it would at least give a truer perspective on the ability of the vaccines to do what their proponents seem to *want* them to do.

I cannot resist pointing out that such research obviously requires a sizable cohort of unimmunized people, which is now being provided by those parents who have refused to immunize their children, despite the concerted efforts of the medical and public health authorities to intimidate and punish them. The same result could of course be achieved much more efficiently by simply making the vaccines *optional*, as they are in West Germany, Sweden, the United Kingdom, and some other places, which would allow the experimental and control groups to select themselves. Our frantic efforts to secure 100 percent compliance with the present mandatory program evidently succeeds only in making such studies impossible.

A closely related type of study would be to measure the effectiveness of *reimmunization* at varying intervals after the original course. In this case, there would be *two* control groups:

1. the same unimmunized cohort, as before; and
2. a group of children previously vaccinated, whose parents decided not to give them a "booster" dose.

This study would also measure the incidence and morbidity of the acute disease when it *does* break out, rather than simply the circulating antibody titer, which is probably far less relevant.

My conjecture, based on the preliminary studies I cited in the text, is that both primary and booster vaccinations tend to give considerably less protection against the corresponding acute disease when it does break out than the simple drop in incidence, or the rise in antibody titer, would indicate.

Both of these studies could also be carried out in suitable animal populations, using vaccines developed against disease peculiar to each species, such as canine distemper, leptospirosis, and the like, inasmuch as what we are concerned with includes the effectiveness and mode of action of the vaccines in general.

A third possibility would be to investigate the relationship between circulating antibody and "immunity" in the above sense. This could be done by measuring antibody titer periodically in a large pooled sample, and then retrospectively comparing baseline titers in an immunized group that subsequently developed the disease with another immunized group that was exposed to the disease but did not develop it. Both could then be compared with the corresponding nonimmunized groups, who would be expected to show no measurable titers at all prior to exposure.

2. How Do the Vaccines Act?

The problem with all of these studies is that they systematically ignore the crucial possibility that the vaccines may act immunosuppressively, and may therefore produce or at least promote a variety of obscure chronic diseases over long periods of time. This is why the "effectiveness" of the vaccines cannot really be studied in isolation without first understanding their mode of action in a more comprehensive fashion.

Indeed, the issue of effectiveness is actually misleading, insofar as it leads us to focus on the typical acute disease, rather than the broad spectrum of biological effects that can be associated with bacteria, viruses, and the vaccines derived from them, a spectrum that includes latent, subclinical, and chronic phenomena as well. We certainly know of situations in which *inability* to develop acute disease represents the exact opposite of good health, i.e., the consequences of chronic immune tolerance rather than true immunity.

At the crudest level, then, we need to study the effects of the vaccines, both acutely and long-term, on various clinical and laboratory parameters of health and disease. In the case of the pertussis vaccine, for example, we need good prospective studies on the incidence and severity of various hematological and CNS abnormalities over time, following the administration of the single vaccine at the usual time (and at routine intervals before and after). This could be done simply and inexpensively by performing CBCs, brief neurological exams, and behavioral assessments on the same self-selected groups of immunized and unimmunized children.

Another method would be to follow certain obvious *clinical* variables at the time of the normal well-child and other pediatric visits, such as the incidence and severity of acute and recurrent URI, tonsillitis, pharyngitis, otitis media, cervical adenopathy, and the like, in both immunized and unimmunized children over a period of years.

The same experimental format should also make it possible to sort out the various patterns of chronic morbidity following each individual vaccine. Again, the crucial importance of the unimmunized cohort becomes obvious. With regard to pertussis, for example, my clinical experience to date strongly suggests that the immunized group will have a significantly higher incidence and morbidity from chronic and recurrent infections, with higher rates of complications and disability, such as myringotomies, hearing loss, etc.

A long-term study could then follow these same children through older childhood and adolescence, to determine the incidence and morbidity of various chronic disease, such as eczema, asthma, rheumatoid arthritis, SLE, ulcerative colitis, multiple sclerosis, and other idiopathic degenerative, CNS, or connective-tissue diseases, as well as mental retardation, hyperactivity, school and behavior problems, convulsive disorders, leukemia, and other forms of cancer. Once again, my suspicion is that the immunized group would show a significantly higher increase in the incidence and morbidity in all these categories. I *hope* I'm wrong, but I don't think I am.

Another interesting and useful study would be to measure the effect of the common vaccines on the incidence and morbidity of other acute infections to which the individual was defintely or probably exposed (influenza, hepatitis, genital herpes, Colorado tick fever, etc.). The point here would be to see if the vaccination process has any effect on the capacity of the immune system to deal with acute infection generally, which seems quite probable.

In this case there would be two control groups:

1. one group of children not previously immunized (against measles, mumps, or whatever), who were subsequently exposed to influenza, hepatitis, or some other acute infection; and
2. a group of similar children who contracted and recovered from acute measles, mumps, or whatever, some time before their exposure to influenza, hepatitis, etc.

Again, my conjecture is that both groups, while perhaps no less likely to *contract* the second disease, would show significantly less acute and chronic *morbidity* as a result of it.

Along these same lines, it would not be very difficult to design some good animal studies investigating the possibility of immunosuppression by the vaccines. This could be done by measuring leukocyte and macrophage activity both in vivo and in vitro, in response to various challenges, such as exposure to unrelated infections, allergens, and chemicals. Various liver function tests, as well as the ability of the spleen and bone marrow to respond to hemorrhage and blood transfusion could also be followed. Finally, the ability of both immunized and un-immunized animals to reject homografts could be measured quite easily.

Careful cytogenetic studies could also be made, to show the effects of vaccination on karyotype and chromosome morphology, beginning with typical "target" cells for which the vaccine in question has a known affinity (e.g., liver parenchymal cells in hepatitis, parotid acinar cells in mumps, cells of the nasal mucosa in measles). Careful virological studies of these same cells should also make it possible to recover or at least demonstrate the existence of episomes or viral nucleoprotein moieties within the DNA or RNA of the host, which would confirm the suspicion of latency and chronic infection, at least in the case of the live vaccine.

But, whichever studies are done, the point is that the technology to do them already exists; and the only thing that prevents them from being done is our own ideological resistance to the self-evident truth that vaccines are not simply "wonder drugs" that produce specific antibodies and nothing more, but complex, biologically active substances whose effects on the human organism urgently need to be investigated.

Notes

1. E. Mortimer, "Pertussis Immunization," *Hospital Practice,* Oct. 1980, p. 103.

2. Quoted in ibid., p. 105.

3. R. Dubos, *Mirage of Health* (Harper, 1959), p. 73.

4. Ibid, pp. 74–75.

5. G. Stewart, "Vaccination Against Whooping Cough: Efficiency vs. Risks," *Lancet,* 1977, p. 234.

6. *Medical Tribune,* 10 Jan. 1979, p. 1.

7. J. Cherry, "The New Epidemiology of Measles and Rubella," *Hospital Practice,* July 1980, pp. 52–54.

8. Private communication from the New Mexico Health Department.

9. M. Lawless, et al., "Rubella Susceptibility in Sixth Graders," *Pediatrics*, 65 (June 1980), pp. 1080–89.

10. Cherry, "Measles and Rubella," p. 53.

11. *Infectious Diseases*, Jan. 1982, p. 21.

12. Cherry, "Measles and Rubella," p. 52.

13. *Family Practice News*, 15 July 1980, p. 1.

14. J. Ferrante, "Atypical Symptoms? It Could *Still* Be Measles," *Modern Medicine*, 30 Sept. 1980, p. 76.

15. Cherry, "Measles and Rubella," p. 53.

16. C. Phillips, "Measles," in V. Vaughan, et al., *Nelson's Textbook of Pediatrics*, 11th ed. (Saunders, 1979), p. 857.

17. B. Davis, et al., *Microbiology*, 2nd ed. (Harper, 1979), p. 1546.

18. Ibid., p. 1346.

19. Ibid., p. 1342.

20. Ibid., p. 1418.

21. L. Hayflick, "Slow Viruses," *Executive Health Report*, Feb. 1981, p. 4.

22. Ibid., pp. 1–4.

23. B. Davis, et al., *Microbiology*, pp. 418–1449.

24. M. Burnet, *The Integrity of the Body* (Atheneum, 1966), p. 4.

25. N. Talai, "Autoimmunity," in Fudenberg, et al., *Basic and Clinical Immunology*, 3rd ed. (Lange, 1980), p. 222.

26. Hayflick, *Slow Viruses*, p. 4.

27. W. McNeill, *Plagues and Peoples* (Anchor, 1976), p. 184.

28. M. Burnet and D. White, *The Natural History of Infectious Disease* (Cambridge, 1976), p. 16.

29. Ibid., pp. 90, 121.

30. A. Steigman, "Slow Virus Infections," in Vaughan, *Nelson's Textbook of Pediatrics*, p. 857.

31. Phillips, "Measles," p. 800.

32. *Infectious Diseases*, April 1979, p. 26.

33. C. Phillips, "Mumps," in Vaughan, *Nelson's Textbook of Pediatrics*, p. 891.

34. G. Hayden, et al., "Mumps and Mumps Vaccine in the U.S.," *Continuing Education*, Sept. 1979, p. 97.

35. Phillips, "Mumps," p. 892.

36. Phillips, "Rubella," p. 863.

37. Ibid., p. 862.

38. L. Glasgow and J. Overall, "Congenital Rubella Syndrome," in Vaughan, *Nelson's Textbook of Pediatrics,* p. 483.

39. Phillips, "Rubella," p. 862.

40. Cited in R. Mendelsohn, "The Truth about Immunizations," *The People's Doctor,* April 1978, p. 1.

41. Stewart, "Whooping Cough," p. 234.

42. Mortimer, "Pertussis Immunization," p. 111.

43. R. Felgin, "Pertussis," in Vaughan, *Nelson's Textbook of Pediatrics,* p. 769.

44. Ibid., p. 769.

45. L. Barnes, "Breast Feeding," in Vaughan, *Nelson's Textbook of Pediatrics,* p. 191.

46. Burnet and White, *Infectious Disease,* p. 91.

47. Davis, et al., *Microbiology,* p. 1290.

48. Ibid., p. 1280.

49. Burnet and White, *Infectious Disease,* p. 93.

50. V. Fulginiti, "Problems of Poliovirus Immunization," *Hospital Practice,* Aug. 1980, pp. 61–62.

51. Burnet and White, *Infectious Disease,* p. 95.

52. Burnet, *The Integrity of the Body,* p. 128.

53. Mendelsohn, "Immunizations," p. 3.

54. Quoted in P. Wehrle, "Vaccines, Risks, and Compensations," *Infectious Diseases,* Feb. 1982, p. 16.

55. Quoted in Mendelsohn, "Immunizations," p. 1.

56. Dubos, *Mirage of Health,* p. 157.

57. T. Kuhn, *The Structure of Scientific Revolutions,* 2nd ed. (Chicago, 1970), chapters 1 and 2.

QUESTION AND ANSWER PERIOD

Q: Why does the American Academy of Pediatrics draft a bill for compensation of vaccine-damaged children that we taxpayers will have to pay for? Why don't the pharmaceutical companies and the doctors and legislators pay for this damage?

Lori Andrews: Before you answer the questions, I'm going to make a suggestion, since I know that the subject of immunization evokes a lot of interest. I wonder if we could get a number of questions and comments first and then you might answer them as a group, and then everybody can have their chance to talk.

Q: How many cases have you found that had cancer developed at the site of the injection? Can you elaborate on Senate Bill S.2117, as to why the taxpayer should not be used to compensate the vaccine-damaged children? In my opinion, epidemics are pharmaceutical clearance sales. Epidemics are seasonal events. All vaccines are iatrogenic. Today's immunized children are tomorrow's asthmatics, diabetics, and cancer victims.

Q: I'd like to make a comment: I recently met a man who had vaccinations 60 years ago. The left half of his body is completely raw and they determined it's all vaccination, just growing in his body. My question is: Since laws on immunizations are enforced more and more, it is our legislators that pass these laws after the lobbyists have talked them into passing the laws. Who are the people who pay the lobbyists to force the immunizations?

Q: Are you familiar at all with John Chris Hofman's work, University of Maryland? He has speculated that vaccine-induced immunity commits more of the body's immune system to that particular antigen, which means they are less available for nonspecific reactions. Have you in your research come across any support for that speculation, and what are your own feelings on that?

Q: I've read some of your other articles on immunizations, and I'd like to know exactly how, in your opinion, a homeopathically prepared remedy would work as opposed· to immunization shots. What is the physiology of what actually takes place biologically?

Q: I'd like to know if you know of any cases where the breast on the opposite side of where the vaccination was to be removed? We know of a lot of them that were on the same side where the vaccine was, but haven't found anybody yet that really had it on the opposite side.

Q: Your talk has been very educational for me, and my question is: What if you refuse shots? I know last year Chicago had a big thing about if you didn't have shots you couldn't get back into the school, and I want to know what options you have if you definitely refuse to have your children vaccinated.

Q: Dr. Moskowitz, from the credits that we heard at the beginning of your speech, I take it that you're not a resident of Illinois, but live in Massachusetts. In response to the question that was just asked—what do parents do for enforced immunizations perpetrated by the school system and the public health authority?—the answer is simple. You have to fight the bastards in court. That's it; it just has to be done that way. I apologize for being so rude, but that, in fact, is the case, because the laws are such that you just have no choice. That's why I think, Dr. Mendelsohn, that immunizations evoke such response from the public, because it is the area in which the freedom of choice of the people is really being taken away from them and they can do very little about it.

Dr. Moskowitz: Maybe I can address some of those questions now. First of all, the lady who asked about cancer at the injection site: No, I have never seen such a thing. It may be possible, but I personally have not seen it or heard of it. In fact, I'd be interested in knowing any documentation you might have of that.

As far as the bill compensating victims of vaccination, I'm opposed to that bill because I think that basically the bill is an attempt to maintain the system as we have it. The American Academy of Pediatrics was challenged by Congress to come up with some guidelines to compensate vaccine-injured people and basically what they came up with is that in order to prove that the victim was injured by the vaccine, they have to show first of all that the effect happened within 30 days of the administration of the vaccine and, secondly, that it has to be an effect that's already been studied or already been discovered. That eliminates immediately the whole concern of my paper, which is precisely those chronic things that happen later, that may be very insidious and very difficult to trace, and for which we as yet have no adequate experimental evidence. So, I think that's a very shortsighted bill and I think really the purpose of it is simply to continue compulsory immunization. I think the bill is paying off a few, a very, very few people, just the very tip of that iceberg there, and the rest of it is being left not only unpaid but uninvestigated as well. That's the whole point of what I'm trying to say, that we need new laws to make those vaccines voluntary. They are in some states; some states have changed the laws in this respect.

As far as the third question goes, I'm not familiar with Dr. Hofman's work, and I'd be very interested in it; but my feeling is that that's only a very small part of what happens because I think the nonspecific immunity is also very important and is probably the reason why measles evolved from a killer disease, which it was at one time. When it was introduced by Cortez into the Americas as the secret weapon of the conquistadores, it decimated whole populations of Mexican villages. It's been estimated to kill about 20 percent of the people infected with it when it meets a population for the first time. The evolution of a disease like measles from a killer into a more or less common disease of childhood which is handled very effectively by the vast majority of people in a population requires generations and generations of what you might call nonspecific or herd immunity, such that when the disease actually strikes, the immune mechanism is already in place waiting for it. So, I think those nonspecific responses are very, very important for the development of what we call true immunity, lifelong immunity, such as you get from recovering from a natural disease.

As far as the homeopathic remedies are concerned, I honestly do not know how the homeopathic remedies work and cannot as yet give you a convincing explanation of how substances as dilute as that can work. We know that they work; we've had the *experience* that they work, and it's a very beautiful, elegant, and safe method. But it implies the existence of a science that in a sense has not been discovered yet, although we're working on it, and trying very hard to elaborate it. I certainly would not say that it's a panacea for every patient with vaccine-related illness, but it certainly can help in many cases.

Someone alluded to the possibility of using a homeopathic remedy in lieu of vaccine. There were homeopaths who advocated that, and indeed there are some people who still do. I myself do not do it because I think the immunization laws are concerned with *long-term* immunity. In order to do that with a homeopathic remedy you would have to give it many, many times, and that's a usage that I would not support. I don't think that long-term immunity is really possible, or even desirable, using artificial means.

As far as the vaccine on the same side as the breast cancer, there again, you've got me; I've never heard of that before. It's very interesting, and I'd like very much to see the information you've collected about it.

As far as the question about the school requirements, I would say that it varies quite a bit from state to state and even from school district to school district. For example, Indiana is one of the many states that, partly in response to public outcry, changed its law so that people may waive the requirement for their children to be immunized if they have a strong philosophical objection to it. They have to sign a waiver that the state gives them; but, even in a state like that, where the law is on the books, to get a school board to allow that may be very difficult. It may take a telephone call from a lawyer or something to let them know that you're really serious to honor the law that exists.

In many other states, in Maryland, for example, the law is quite rigid and without exception: There are no exceptions, except in some cases, if the doctor writes a letter of exemption for very strong medical reasons, such as for a child who has a high fever or convulsions at the time of the test. In that case everyone would agree that the immunization should not be given. If there was a strong history of neurological disease, they might also entertain such a letter; but this whole area that we were getting into here about the connection between vaccines and chronic disease would not be allowed at present in a state such as Maryland.

HOSPITAL BIRTHS

A Dissenting View

Gregory White, M.D.

INTRODUCTION OF THE SPEAKER

Lori Andrews: Over the past day and a half, we've been moving toward examples of dissent that are increasingly in the public eye. We talked initially about some areas of health care in which there was dissent within the medical profession, but I think the area of immunization and the subject of Dr. Gregory White's discussion today on hospital births vs. home births are areas of dissent about which more and more people are aware. People are trying to gain access to rights of choice about whether or not to submit to these procedures.

With the growing public recognition of the dissent, though, has come a high cost to the practitioners involved. I know that in the home birth area, practitioners who have offered this option have run into problems such as their malpractice insurance being revoked or their hospital backup privileges being revoked.

To discuss in greater detail today a dissenting view of hospital births, we will hear from Dr. Gregory White, who is the president of the American College of Home Obstetrics, has a family practice in Franklin Park, Illinois, and was an undergraduate at Loyola University, where he also obtained his medical degree. Dr. White is a senior staff member at Westlake Hospital in Melrose Park, and at Loretto Hospital he serves as president elect of the medical staff. He's the author of *Emergency Childbirth*.

LECTURE

Dr. White: I've had some personal experience, family experience, with birth as well as professional experience. I did do hospital births for 40 years until about a year ago. My hospital privileges in obstetrics, family practice level, were revoked because, along with two other family practitioners, I refused to give up home births. But, as I say, I have personal experience as well. My wife and I had our first three babies in the hospital and our last eight babies at home. Twenty-one of my 23 grandchildren have been born at home, so my high opinion of home birth is more than theoretical. There's been a lot of criticism of the medical profession at this conference, all of it richly deserved, and you're going to hear some more in a few minutes, but first I would like to state that I am proud and happy to be a member of the medical profession. Why is that? Because we're rich and powerful? No, we aren't. Because we're learned? No. I think we deserve your respect for being learned, but never underestimate the ignorance of a learned man—especially when your life or your health is at stake. (Never underestimate your own ignorance, either. Humility is something all of us need in the profession and out of it.) But I'm proud to be a doctor and I'm proud to be a brother of other doctors, and that does include even obstetricians and neonatologists. I'm proud to be a physician because we do spend our lives caring for others. Most of my brother and sister physicians are more selfless than they get credit for.

The conflict we're seeing at this conference is in large part a fight between the tradition of Hippocrates, a great physician who practiced several hundred years before Christ and who taught humility to physicians, humility in the face of the subtlety and complexity of nature, and the "American Way." Hippocrates taught the value of medical learning not for its own sake but for the patient's sake. He taught physicians to practice in cooperation with nature and to teach the patient. This is where the word doctor comes from; it means *teacher*. Hippocrates taught the patient to cooperate with nature. He taught that when we're confronted with an illness, we turn first to regimen—in other words, diet—and exercise, rest, and if necessary, changes in life-style. If that isn't enough, then we add medicines, and if that isn't enough, as a final treatment, surgery in certain cases.

This priority is violated far too often today, as has been said by others here. The Hippocratic tradition came down to us through Western

Europe, a rather settled part of the world, although they had their wars and their famines and all the usual things disturbing them. But there was continuity, a conservative village way of life. I met a man a few years ago, Dr. William Mercer Daley of Dublin, a very fine physician who had twelve generations of physicians behind him. Now, this is something we can hardly even imagine in America. You can imagine what a rich tradition there is in that one family. This conservative, cooperative view of medicine has come down to us in this country, too. It's alive and well today as witnessed by Dr. Bob Mendelsohn. Hippocrates is worth reading, but you need a guide as you do when you read Dante. He's a total mystery to most physicians, including myself, without such a guide. I recommend that you read something about him by Dr. Herbert Ratner, who knows him well.

But we came to this country (our ancestors did at any rate) and things changed. The old mottos like "Look before you leap" were changed to things like "He who hesitates is lost," and if the new settler was confronted by a wild bear or an Indian shooting arrows at him, he who hesitated *was* lost. We physicians are part of our culture; we're in it with all the rest of you. The epitome of American physicians was Benjamin Rush. One of the medical schools here in Chicago is named after him. He was a signer of the Declaration of Independence, he was an army surgeon in the Revolution, and he was an authentic hero. He stayed in Philadelphia during the yellow fever epidemic and treated patients until he reached the point of exhaustion. When other doctors were running out of town to escape infection, he stayed and caught the fever. But his treatments were as heroic as his career. He purged them and puked them and bled them, and if they died it was the disease and if they survived it was the treatment. He had the same things done to himself when he got yellow fever. He was a therapeutic enthusiast and he felt that diseases could be conquered just like George III's "lobster backs" could be conquered.

As I said, the old tradition has persisted, too. Some of you have read Oliver Wendell Holmes, Sr., professor of Harvard Medical School, father of the famous jurist and codiscoverer with Semmelweis of the cause and prevention of puerperal or childbed fever. He even wrote about laetrile, believe it or not, back in the 1840s and 1850s. (They called it amygdalin then.) He taught us some conservatism. He reacted against the tradition of Benjamin Rush, but the frontier moved on anyway.

Men were men, and women were scarce and they had no time to be midwives because they were all married and raising families of their own and, besides that, the conditions of the frontier made the male virtues predominant in delivering babies. What are the manly strengths? We all know what a woman's strengths are, but a man is a bit bigger, he's a bit stronger physically, he can be at times a little bit faster moving. The physician could hop on a horse and ride through a blizzard 40 miles to deliver a baby, while sometimes the midwife wouldn't make it if the snow was too deep. And there weren't many midwives. We got out of the tradition of midwives which is so powerful in Europe. There are a few midwives still, and there are more coming, but in America birth was turned over to the male doctor, whose gifts for getting to the birth— strength and activism—became drawbacks when he arrived.

Now, obstetrics was in horrible condition in the early 1930s; our maternal death rate was one of the worst of the developed nations, an international scandal. A lot of people made studies of the causes—we'll get into some of those—and a lot of them made recommendations (most of which were not followed). Gradually, due to the old death fighters like Dr. Joseph DeLee, who taught in this city, and Dr. Greenhill, his successor, who taught me in medical school, and my other teachers, this improved. These men were death fighters. Safety was not the first or the last consideration; it was the only consideration. They didn't care what they did to mothers or babies as long as they brought them through alive. To some degree, this is the bottom line, but to ruin birth for millions of women and their babies, to get them off to a very bad start on their mothering and their family living in order to save one or two, may be a bad trade-off.

At any rate, home birth, which had been fashionable in this country, was the only way of birth through most of the world up to and including the present time. Most of the people in the world, 3½ billion or more of them, have been born in one-room cabins, attended by a midwife who may or may not have had some training. The reproductive process on the whole is pretty successful or there wouldn't be so many people around.

Home births started to go out of fashion in the United States; by 1935 only half of American babies were born at home. From 1935 on, there was a steady decline until about 1980, and at the same time the maternal mortality rate went way down. The obstetricians said, "See, the maternal mortality rate has gone down because the home birth rate has gone down." Well, it's not true. That's an old error in logic known as *"post hoc ergo propter hoc,"* meaning, "after which therefore because of which." If Dr. Mendelsohn walks out of the room and this chandelier falls on all the people under it, that doesn't mean he caused it just because the one event preceded the other.

The things that reduced the maternal mortality rate most were brought out in the early forties when we got antibiotics and blood banks. Two main causes of maternal death were infection and hemorrhage. Toxemia was the third. We've discovered how to prevent that through diet and how to treat it with the new drugs that we have now. So, the three killers in childbirth have been to a large degree conquered and the improvement in mortality has been just as great for home births as it has been for hospital births.

Now, there are many papers demonstrating the safety of home birth and I certainly can't give you the details on all of them, but I would like to recommend to you two books which summarize and can make you a really informed person on home and hospital birth. One is *Home Birth* by Dr. Stanley Sagov, an Aspen publication, and the other is *The Place of Birth*, edited by Sheila Kitzinger and John Davis, Oxford University Press. There have been a number of studies that demonstrated just the opposite of what they were expected to from the early thirties on. The New York Academy of Medicine between 1930 and 1932 made an extensive study of births in the New York area and found to their horrified astonishment that home was safer than the hospital, that midwives were safer than doctors, and that among the doctors family practitioners were safer than obstetricians. This is not a comparison of all cases because obstetricians do handle the tough ones but a comparison of obstetricians vs. family practitioners in low-risk cases. The Frontier Nursing Service in Kentucky in the poorest part of Appalachia went back into the hills and delivered undernourished women in hovels from 1925 to the late sixties and had an excellent safety record, much better than the national average. These were trained nurse midwives. They were working with what they could carry on their backs or in the saddlebags of a horse in the early years, or in a jeep in later years, and they did good work. In North Carolina in 1974 and 1976, the Center for Disease Control in Atlanta made a study of births and found that midwives were better and home births were better.

We had a saying when I was in medical school (it sounds very sexist but it's really not). It tells you more about the art than it does about the difference betweeen men and women. The saying was, "Women make good obstetricians; they're not strong enough to be bad obstetricians." As I say, that tells you a lot about the art. In the delivery rooms at Lying

In Hospital they used to have mottos on the wall; they may be there yet. One was "Not force but art *(Non vi sed arte)*," and the other was "First do no harm *(Primum non nocere)*."

These sayings are from the heritage of Hippocrates and Western European medicine. They are contradicted in large part by our horrifying 22 percent national rate of cesarean sections. It's probably higher than that by now, but that was the last reported figure. There are still hospitals with a 2 to 5 percent cesarean rate which are demonstrating very low perinatal mortality—that is the mortality of babies before, during, and after birth. But there are still other places that are up to 40 and 50 percent section rates. Now, a cesarean section, according to all papers that have ever been written on the subject, is about 10 times as risky to the mother's life and about 30 times as risky to her health as natural birth.

Thank God we have the operation for the 1 to 2 percent of women who really need cesarean sections. It's a great operation, but like every other bit of technology in American medicine, it's been overused. The same goes for a great many other things that we have in American medicine like ultrasound, which has its place—a very small place, and maybe it'll vanish eventually, but it does make diagnoses that we can't otherwise make in a few pathological cases. However, there are doctors using it in their offices so that mothers can see the fetuses move. This is a great sentimental pleasure to the mother, but they don't know what the risk is to the baby. There may be a risk, there may not. Animal experiments suggest it might be harmful. We do know that some risks are worth taking if you get a payoff benefit from taking those risks, but we're taking risks without comparable benefits in too many cases.

I would like to tell you about a study that Dr. Lewis Mehl made in 1976 of 1,046 mothers at home and 1,046 comparable mothers in the hospital. These women were pretty well matched for age, parity and social class, factors which have bearing on health. I'm not going to give you the results, which were in favor of the home birth group—that is, the babies had fewer sicknesses and fewer problems, as did the mothers too in the home groups—but I just want to contrast what was done at home and in the hospital.

These two groups were compared very carefully. In the first stage, Pituitrin or oxytocin was used to stimulate labor in about 69 of the 1,046 home births and in 159 of the 1,046 hospital births. During the second stage of labor, labor was stimulated by Pitocin (oxytocin) in 38 cases at home and 159 cases in the hospital. In the third stage of labor, after the baby was born, and when the placenta was coming, the uterus was stimulated by Pitocin at home in 251 cases, and in the hospital, in 993. Outlet forceps at home: 3 out of 1,046, 115 at the hospital. Cesarean sections (remember this was 1976): 28 people who had been scheduled for home births (these weren't done at home, of course, but all complications that took place in the patients that had originally been scheduled for home delivery and transferred to the hospital were referred back to the home birth group; otherwise, it would be an unfair comparison entirely), but 28 sections in the home group, and 86 among the hospital group. Today that would probably be around 200 or 300 in the hospital group if it were an average American group. Fourth-degree laceration of the perineum: five at home, 73 in the hospital. Cervical lacerations: three at home, 32 in the hospital. Why?—interference (the high forceps rate and so forth). Analgesia (drugs to relieve pain): in the home 14 out of 1,046 mothers, in the hospital 555 out of 1,046 mothers. Pudendal anesthesia (injection of Novocain into certain nerves in a woman's pelvis): none at home, 655 in the hospital. General (gas) anesthesia: 2 in the home group, although these had been transferred to the hospital, and 96 in the hospital group. Paracervical block (an injection in the nerves around the cervix or the uterus): 1 in the home group, and 52 in the hospital.

That they were doing so much more in the hospital explains in large part why home birth is safer. Home birth is safer bacteriologically, but that's a very minor factor. The woman in her own home is immune to the germs that are in her home. If the birth attendant who comes in is careful about his or her cleanliness, the mother is safe. The woman in the hospital delivers in a room where three other women may have delivered in the same day. That means there have been two other doctors besides hers in there, there have been three shifts of nurses, residents, cleaning ladies, etc. This is why we must be fanatical about sterility in the hospital. This is why three babies are dead in Maryland, according to the last *AMA News*, because of a hospital nursery epidemic. Five babies were affected, three died. You can't get that kind of an epidemic in a home where there's one mother and one baby (barring the occasional case of twins). The main factor of risk in the hospital, though, is not infection. The main factor is that the doctor feels that with the hospital enveloping him and backing him up he is free to go ahead and do anything that he's been trained to do.

The first operation that an obstetric resident does is an episiotomy, and every obstetrician takes pride in the fact that his episiotomies heal a little more quickly and with less pain than any other doctor's episiotomies. Just ask them sometime when they've had a couple of drinks, and they'll tell you all about it. I can regard this with sympathy, at least. I remember when I was a young resident assisting a delivery in a small community hospital, and an elderly family practitioner was there with his patient. He was probably not as old as I am now, but I was the smart, young resident and this woman, of course, was flat on her back with her legs up in the stirrups. It was her first baby, it was an occiput posterior, she had started pushing, and we were all gowned and gloved. The heart tones got slow and a bit irregular and, with the permission of the attending physician, I grabbed my trusty DeLee forceps and did a mid-forceps rotation very slickly and quickly (the Bill modification of the Scanzoni maneuver for those of you who are technically minded), and hauled out a screaming kid. The old family practitioner pounded me on the back and the young, good-looking female intern looked admiringly at me, and the nurses said, "Oh, doctor, you saved that baby's life." What would I do nowadays with a case like that? Well, I'd get the woman out of the stirrups, and turn her on her side, and probably the heart tones would improve. I might even give her a little oxygen. But midwives can do that; that's not dramatic; that's not any exhibition of technical skill. It might have an equally good result for the baby, but you can see how we get hooked on what we do, and on our skills and on what we've learned, and it takes a long time to unlearn some things.

The coverage of home births in the medical literature of the United States has been limited. We do have papers indicating safer home births than hospital births in low-risk cases. But this has really been tested abroad, especially in Holland. For many years Dr. G. J. Kloosterman, who was Professor of Obstetrics, now Emeritus, at the University of Amsterdam and who had charge of the home birth service for all of Holland, has written extensively on the safety of home birth. He told me a couple of years ago that the perinatal mortality rate in home births in Holland is one-third that of low-risk hospital births.

Why don't obstetricians listen? Why don't they read these statistics? Why aren't they impressed by them? Because it goes contrary to everything they've been taught to believe—and again we're up against beliefs. If you'd ask an obstetrician about home birth, nine times out of ten either you'll get a horror story about some woman who died on the front steps of his hospital because she had attempted a home birth or he will say, "Well, what if this happens, or what if that happens?" But there have been thousands of cases studied to demonstrate the safety of home birth. The occasional weird case doesn't prove one thing, whether it's in the hospital or in the home.

And, of course, if it's in the home, it's "criminal malpractice." I know one doctor who was charged with murder for delivering a baby at home. The baby later died in the hospital, although he'd gotten the baby there in pretty good condition and the baby was there for 19 hours being subjected to every treatment known to man before it died. Some of the treatments may have been necessary. The doctor who took care of the baby in the hospital was charged with nothing, and that doctor wrote on the baby's admission, "The baby is pink, vigorous, and crying." That sounds pretty good to me. That doesn't sound like a dying baby.

At any rate, doctors and midwives are being driven out of practice across the country from coast to coast, from here to Canada. They are losing their licenses, they are being accused of manslaughter, murder, you name it. They are being vilified, they are being lied about, they are being smeared. What does the future hold? Well, we need more midwives and we need more home births, and we need less intervention in hospital births. But we're not likely to get these things unless an informed and aroused lay public demands them.

QUESTION AND ANSWER PERIOD

Dr. White: Rick Moskowitz, veteran of home births, wants to talk.

Dr. Moskowitz: I just wanted to make a comment, Greg. I did home births for 13 years myself and I just have a feeling that part of the problem with hospital birth is simply one of scheduling, too. As a home birth person, basically what I have to offer is myself, my energy, my presence, plus the midwife who's there with me, so that means I can do about four births a month, maybe, in addition to everything else I do. A busy hospital-based obstetrician with the monitors and everything can usually do about 30 births a month, and if you're responsible for that number of births, you just have to see that they get through there really fast; you can't wait for somebody to just go through labor and do it. You've got to crank them out of there, you know.

Dr. White: This is why Northwestern University closed the Chicago Maternity Center home delivery service. The residents are looking for technical experience, and a big day for a home birth resident, a very big day indeed, would be three births. If the resident is in the hospital, he or she can do several times that number of births. At County Hospital they call it "the labor line"; they'll say, "She's 'on the line,'" meaning she's in labor. This is an assembly line, there are no bones about it. The resident can crank out eight or 10 births in an ordinary working day, and he or she gets a lot more technical experience, a lot more episiotomies done and repaired, a lot more chances to use forceps. This is what he or she is a resident for, to learn surgical techniques. The professors of obstetrics said they couldn't get residents for the home birth service, so they closed it. At least that's one of the main reasons they closed it.

Susan Dart: Dr. Crile said yesterday, I believe I'm quoting him correctly, that there are three unnecessary operations that soon, he thought (I think, hope) would not be done anymore. He named tonsillectomies, mastectomies, and circumcisions. I wonder if you could give us a medical justification for circumcision.

Dr. White: There is none. There are no medical justifications for circumcisions. I have no objection to it as a religious ceremony but as a medical procedure it's nonsense.

Q: Dr. White, I can't keep my mouth shut. My training was from Great Britain and I had done home births before, and, when I first came to this country in 1965 and worked at Chicago Maternity Center, I enjoyed it tremendously up until the time when I went back and practiced in the hospital. Our protocol was that we could use Demerol up to 75 milligrams for . . . the routine episiotomy and so on. Then, when I went back to Baltimore, the midwives all came and asked me, "Would you help with the home births?" And I would say to the mother, "Well, what baby is this?" She would say "This is my first baby." I said, "Well, we may have to do an episiotomy," and they objected, so I said to myself, "Why not try and help them the way they want?" and from that day forward I have never done one single episiotomy. That was in 1974. And there's no such thing as having to put the mother up on the stirrups. I found when I went on the home births that mothers can be in any position they want: If they want to squat that's fine; if they want to stand and have the baby that way, that's fine.

Dr. White: A woman is queen in her own home. She has something to say about her choices, and in a hospital she has almost nothing to say about them. It's wonderful that you're letting her make her own personal decisions.

All of us who do home births try to be quiet. We don't want to end up in jail, but it's a little difficult. About 10 days ago a woman called me from Canada and asked if I would do a home birth at a friend's house here in Chicago and I said, "Why do you want to come down here?," and she said, "I had a home birth in Canada three years ago and now the doctor is not allowed to deliver babies at home or in the hospital. He's out of obstetric practice. The midwives up here were going to take my case but they've now refused because my baby is breech. I've been to five different obstetricians asking for natural birth, and all of them have said, 'Well, we'll see how it goes. Maybe we won't do a cesarean, but of course you'll have stirrups and an episiotomy and forceps to the aftercoming head and anesthesia.' " And she said, "I don't want those things" and they said, "Sorry, look somewhere else for care." So she called me and I couldn't promise her a thing, but I said, "If you want to come down, I'll examine you and we'll see what's what. So she did and everything was fine. The baby was small; it was a frank breech. I went to her friend's home. The mother was in active labor and very shortly, in front of the student whom I was prepared to initiate into the mysteries of the maneuvers of delivering a breech, the baby came out. I was gowned, gloved, and ready, and the baby plopped out and that was it. I had no chance to even lay a hand on the child.

Dr. Moskowitz: I just wanted to add one other benefit of home birth which is implicit. Instead of being in the guise of telling a patient what to do or what is best for her, the doctor becomes the servant of the patient; the doctor is assisting the patient in her own process. The doctor is simply being there in whatever capacity he can, and the patient is calling the shots. The patient is sharing the responsibility with the doctor. The doctor or the midwife or whomever is simply helping. So the relationship of the midwife, to me, is a prototype of the doctor-patient relationship in a holistic setting.

Dr. White: When I'm in the home, I'm a guest; when I'm in the hospital, the patient is the subject, you might say. It's a big difference.

CLOSING REMARKS

Lori Andrews: Thank you, Dr. White. I think all of the speakers this morning in one way or another have alluded to the effects of the laws, and I'd like to briefly touch upon why the laws have gotten to the point where they seem in many instances counterproductive. With the specific questions on the immunization laws, these laws are really antiquated. The statutes were passed 100 years ago. At that time the U.S. Supreme Court upheld the states' right to require immunizations. The Court felt that mandatory vaccinations, like a mandatory draft, were necessary to protect the public. The Court believed that it was too dangerous to allow the possibility of an unvaccinated child passing on an illness to others. Today, however, there is a need to reassess these laws. Looking at it now, we can legitimately ask how much a risk of contagion there is today. Even if there is some risk along those lines, shouldn't it be something that we as a society tolerate so that people can have their choices?

The law has also been very concerned with risk in the home birth area as well. Some lawmakers want to prohibit midwives from performing a home birth because they fear the midwives would not be able to recognize that small percentage of births—say, 10 percent—where a home birth was not appropriate and there was a risk. I think the studies along those lines are very gratifying. They show that midwives are very competent at turning over to physicians and hospitals those women who are at higher risk.

The law is extremely quick to analyze the risks of alternatives to physicians. I'd like to argue at this point for a change in the approach of the laws to try to look at the risks of some of the traditional and authorized procedures. As was pointed out today, there are risks with vaccination that may be lingering in our bodies and have profound effects in the years to come. There are risks in hospital births, and one of the biggest risks which was alluded to is the cascade of interventions. Once there's one intervention, a labor-inducing drug given, it's far more likely that the next intervention will take place, that there would be a cesarean section, that there would be pain killers given, and so on, with increased risk to the infant and mother at each step of the way. So, I'm hoping that this conference and others like it will help refocus the laws on the real risks and benefits in medicine today.

Dr. Mendelsohn: I'd like to list the major characteristics of this meeting very quickly. The first is that it represents a meeting of doctors and people, and for me that's a very unusual experience. I think that it's been demonstrated that, to at least some degree, doctors can talk to people and people can talk to doctors in the kind of language that both groups can understand.

Secondly, we've had doctors from a variety of age groups, and we've had doctors from a great variety of practices—from full-time academic work to private practice and everything in between. These nine dissenters—I call them that with apologies to Dr. Henry Heimlich, who says that the other side are dissenters and we are not—represent just a fraction of all the dissenters. Because when we made up the list, we were capable of coming up with twenty or thirty easily.

The third characteristic is that truths were heard today that are not commonly heard either at medical meetings or at meetings of lay audiences, and I think that's significant.

The fourth characteristic is that the meeting was held within the medical establishment. That's why we decided to call the meeting "Dissent in Medicine." Not that the dissent outside of medicine is not important, but that's what we chose as the boundaries for this meeting.

The next characteristic is that this meeting was held at very low expense, comparatively speaking, because this should be a fifty thousand-dollar meeting as far as funding is concerned. But because all the speakers came without receiving a fee, and most of them came without receiving expenses, and because James Chatz, chairman of the board of the foundation, provided his leadership without pay, and because Mort

Kaplan did the public relations without pay, we were able to run, what I would suggest is a first meeting of its kind—and I hope not the only one of its kind—with very little expense.

Next is that when I listen to people like Dr. Spodick and Dr. Crile, I think to myself that when anybody wants to look for nominees for the next head of the FDA or the Surgeon General's office, those are the kind of people who should be in the running.

The next characteristic is that the underlying single theme of this meeting, if I'm correct, is the challenge to all of us to ask for controlled scientific studies. Not to downplay the importance of anecdotal reports, but for those of you who are interested in science, I would suggest that that's a common denominator.

The next characteristic is the interest people have in this kind of meeting. Yesterday we had over 250 people in this room, and today I did a quick count and almost 200 came back. I regard that as significant, since these meetings were held on weekdays.

Next is that there were a variety of consumer groups represented here, some of whom you saw yesterday represented by their officers and a number of whom are represented today.

The next is that even though this meeting did not specifically address itself to the economics of medicine, I think that economics ran through every presentation. I think that if the recommendations of the nine speakers were carried out, the cost of medical care would probably drop about 90 percent. I have a feeling that the only way there will ever be a rational basis for reducing the cost of medical care will be to tell people, as we've tried to do here both yesterday and today, about the futility of most of medical treatment and the danger of medical treatment so that medical treatment may be freely available but nobody will apply for it.

The next characteristic that this meeting demonstrated was that technology works. I'm referring specifically to the presentation by video of Dr. Ed Pinkney, who wasn't able to be with us. This may set an example for future meetings of this kind, if they are ever held.

I'd like to thank all of you who attended today, thank all of the speakers, the media who attended and who are really our microphone to the world, and everyone who is responsible for implementing the many details that went into this meeting—which, as the speakers know, was just initiated about two and a half months ago. I'd like to thank the three moderators who helped keep things running smoothly, and disciplined doctors, a group notoriously hard to discipline. Thank you very much.

The *Dissent in Medicine* meeting upon which this book is based is one of the activities of the New Medical Foundation, a tax-exempt organization designed to support innovative forms of medical education of the public and the medical profession. Contributions are welcome to help support and expand the Foundation's activities and may be mailed to:

> James A. Chatz
> Chairman of the Board
> The New Medical Foundation
> 36th Floor
> 115 South LaSalle Street
> Chicago, IL 60603

Also by Robert S. Mendelsohn, M.D., from Contemporary Books:

Confessions of a Medical Heretic (1979; paperback by Warner Books)
Male Practice: How Doctors Manipulate Women (1981; paperback 1982)
How to Raise a Healthy Child in Spite of Your Doctor (1984)

Dr. Mendelsohn also publishes a monthly subscription newsletter, *The People's Doctor Newsletter* (P.O. Box 792, Evanston, Illinois 60204), and writes a syndicated newspaper column (Columbia Features, New York).

INDEX

DATE DUE			
April 14, 2010			
MAY 12 1988			

DEMCO 38-297